The InterGalactic Café

The InterGalactic Café

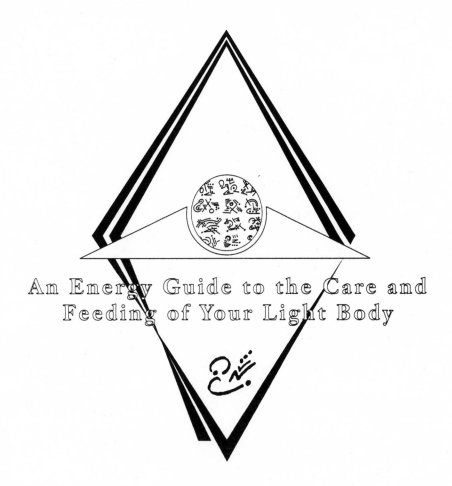

An Energy Guide to the Care and Feeding of Your Light Body

zho-de-Rah and Zon-O-Ray

SAMUEL WEISER, INC.

York Beach, Maine

First published in 2001 by
Samuel Weiser, Inc.
P. O. Box 612
York Beach, ME 03910-0612
www.weiserbooks.com

Library of Congress Cataloging-in-Publication Data
(Available from the Library of Congress upon request.)

ISBN 1-57863-226-9

Typeset in 9/13 Americana

Front cover and all artform symbologies by Zon-O-Ray
Book design and editing by zho-de-Rah

Printed in the United States of America
VG

07 06 05 04 03 02 01
9 8 7 6 5 4 3 2 1

The paper used in this publication meets the minimum requirements
of the American National Standard for Information Sciences—
Permanence of Paper for Printed Library
Materials Z39.48-1992 (R1997).

◦ Dedication ◦

It has been said that some are born to greatness
while others simply have it thrust upon them.

This book is the culmination of all our researches which conclude
that **all** are born to greatness and this greatness
is right now being thrust upon us all.

And so this book is dedicated to all those
great light bodies now emerging.
This is chart topping, heart stopping stuff.
And so we say "C'mon guys, let's rock 'n' roll
outta the night right into that light!
Yah ! "

Contents

∘ Introduction ∘

This book contains one simple idea, that inside every
human body is a light body wanting to get out.

If you're in any way worried about this light body thing,
rest assured. You've got one all right. Every body does.

If somehow you mislaid your instruction book for it, relax.
It's all encoded in your DNA anyway.

That new life you ordered has now arrived.
All you have to do is unwrap it.
What's more, it's free.

The moment you've been waiting ages for is here.
You were born to ascend into a faster and higher
vibrational aspect of yourself,
Light Body.

And the time is now.

◦ Your Spiritual Directions ◦
also known as IN◦sights

What we share with you in these pages is
what worked for us.

Each being is unique
with a unique aspect of The plan encoded.
We share our data not as the one and only truth
but as stimulation to your own truth, that inner knowing
of who you are, why you are here,
and what is yours to do.

Please read this book in this spirit,
with whom it has been written.

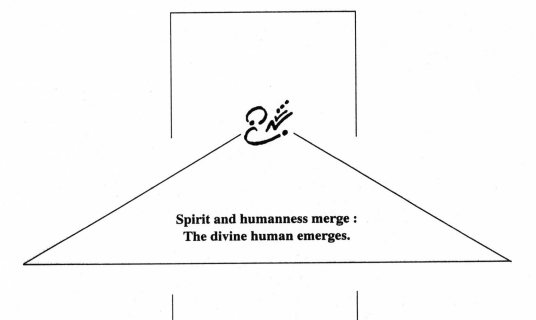

Spirit and humanness merge :
The divine human emerges.

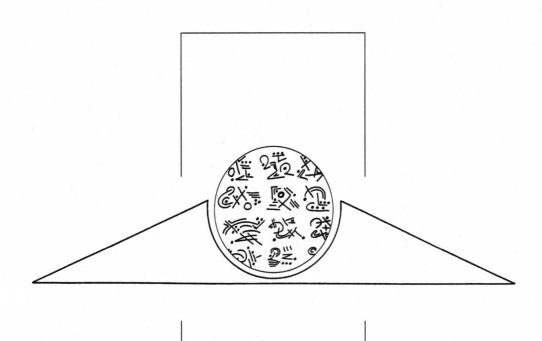

The Origins of the InterGalactic Café

The Set Up

If anyone had told me that I'd be preparing food for 15 or so people twice a day for 3 or 4 months I would have said they were nuts. Formerly I really would only cook when I felt like it. Well, so much for that one. However unwilling or untrained for this job I may have felt, the more I got into it the more apparent it was that I was totally knowledgeable somewhere else. It was truly amazing.

Mighty oaks from little acorns grow, as we all know. And so it all began innocuously enough with my offer to make lunch each day for a friend who could never find time for it. Very quickly the name arrived, **The InterGalactic Café**. Everyone thought it was really fun and loved the name. Along with the name came many more people. In the two months or so leading up to all this, when I was experimenting in my kitchen "laboratory" for 6 to 7 hours at a stretch and still baking at 2 am, Zon asked me what I was doing. *I'm not quite sure,* I said, *but it feels like I'm feeding millions.* Little did I know.

Clarity dawned as more and more pieces of the jigsaw began to fall into place. It quickly became apparent that the Café was part of something much larger, **The InterGalactic Clinic**. Our little programme here on Earth with a handful of galactic representatives was feeding data, vibrationally, to those millions of beings I had so clearly sensed.

So, there we were, diving straight into the gene pool of this planet and with that, many many others of its off-planet seeding systems besides. It was a blast.

One day it all abruptly stopped. I just knew I wouldn't be doing it anymore. What happened? A few days later I began writing what you're now reading, **food for thought**.

We feel that quite an important purpose has been served through the learning curve of this project. As a result of it, we find ourselves living demonstrations of a whole new way of living, being and doing as part of what is now emerging for everyone else on the planet. Everyone can, and will, do **their thing**. You can hardly avoid that since everyone carries their mission in their genes too. It's as natural to express that now as intergalactic apple pie.

So, if our experiences or anything in this book set some of those wheels in motion for you, we're glad that this purpose has been served.

Enter The Players

It has been said that inside every fat person is a thin one wanting to get out. This focuses attention on one's appearance, or health, or both. The events of the recent past have led me to a whole new conclusion which is this :

> **Inside each human being is a whole new divine**
> **galactic being actually coming out**

When our early ancestors the dinosaurs had fulfilled their purpose and were ready to move to their next step, they simply transformed into our present day birds. What is happening to humans is this : our next phase is now being triggered for the leap into light body.

Life Force guides this process. It takes the form of cosmic rays or radiations. These intelligent light forms call our present life force forms into their higher resonant frequency. They electromagnetically feed our etheric bodies and subsequently our physical bodies. Some call this en-light-enment. Some at-one-ment. Some ascension. Some descension of spirit into matter. Whatever you may call it, these are just various expressions of one and the same thing. In this new life form, spirit is the motive force.

The Life Force guiding this process is able to be assimilated and integrated into the body via live organic foods. Chlorophyll is constituted the same as blood is. In the human body chlorophyll actually becomes blood, fixing and carrying new cosmic energies or frequencies into the cellular data banks, the DNA. These frequencies of the cosmic mind field and the DNA code talk a bit together. The new data streams through the physical, mental and emotional body energy fields as they fine tune the light body to come on line.

Frequency modulators, or low frequency level matrices, which have held the dense physical body in its current shape for so long are now being released. With that release, the long dormant 99% of your so far unused DNA and the 90% of unused brain capacity come on line. Concomitantly this current reality shape shifts and slowly dematerializes as the new one makes its appearance. You can't take any form from within a density field into the new light field. This is what is meant by "you can't take it with you."

What is required of all of us is this : to see the new way that it is as it makes its appearance and focus on that, rather than trying to turn back the clock and hang on to things in the old way that it was.

This quotation from *Illusions* by Richard Bach drawing from the force of Nature is a wonderfully apt summary of where we're at :

> **What the caterpillar calls a death**
> **the Master calls a butterfly ***

---

* New York: Dell, 1989.

Highlights of the Plan

Biogenetic Food

Raw organic foods are biogenetic. Plants contain cosmic life force so humanity can ingest the evolutionary forces of Nature they carry. The part these intelligent beings play is the purposeful co-creation of Heaven on Earth with us. They also carry the oldest and most enduring life forms on Earth. For the mineral and rock kingdom is cheering us on too.

Over the last few months of this big little intergalactic project, I have developed the habit of giving a little prayer of thanks to these beings for their contributions. It is in fact thanks to these life streams that human consciousness opens a little more each day. They open and pave the way for the gifts of spirit, our spiritual essence, to reside more deeply within us, every day in every way. Thanks guys.

The InterGalactic Food Programme

We were guided to use the aptly titled *Fit For Life* principles brought through by the two Diamonds, Marilyn and Harvey.* Thank you guys. This observes and catalyzes the body's three 8 hour cycles :

Intake	:	Noon to 8 PM
Integrate	:	8 PM to 4 AM
Eliminate	:	4 AM to Noon

Fresh, raw, organic fruit and/or juice is eaten before noon. Lunch and dinner primarily consist of a salad along with something a little heavier and sustaining which is usually cooked, followed frequently, but not always, with a small sweet treat. Everyone on the programme was working and they all reported easy digestion, loads more energy and no bloating or fullness.

Many different foods have been seeded here by our off-planet ancestors contributing to humanity's transition. Different genetics require different vibrations to activate. Different strokes for different folks. So the meals are not vegetarian or dairy free. We used raw unpasteurized milk free of bovine growth hormone (rBGH).

In following spirit, your inner awareness hooks up to access your vaster knowing or the cosmic mind field. This is way beyond the **thinking** knowing of a mind conditioned by human limitation and personal wants and dislikes. So this is what is really going on beneath what merely seems to be going on.

There was no choice. Everyone ate what arrived and loved it. It was not until I came to write this book that I suddenly noticed how subtle and powerful were the choices the other dimensional teams made. You will see from the menu and recipe sections that many of the foods hark back to "ancient" times. To maximize the cosmic vibrations being anchored in the food, the receiving and transmission powers of the hands were used.

Living Genetic Synergies

Once the maximum number of the "representatives" on this program was reached, it remained fairly constant. However what I see looking at it now is this. There was clearly a core or nucleus of people around whom revolved various "electrons," so to speak. These electrons came, stayed awhile, and then departed to be replaced at certain intervals. It seems so obvious now in this atomic context, that a living, breathing, energetically structured genetic and molecular synergy came in to play.

Over time word spread about this food programme. Many people wanted to join and it became very clear that certain energetics and genetics were to participate. I just naturally found myself evolving into doing a scanning process to identify mission members of this project. You see, a mission is not a business. It's an enterprise with a spiritual directive. Ours serves and supports transubstantiation processes, the transition from density to light body.

This InterGalactic Café and Clinic is a light infusion mission. It is guided totally by spiritual forces and our other dimensional teams or forces. Our prices and our work follow this lead by spirit. In the new world we're poised to enter, what we do and our resources are not co-dependent as has been the norm on Earth and which is now passing away.

Because the food was unusual, someone asked me to write down for them what was in each meal. And so, fortuitously, we now have the menu and recipe sections of this book. I think the teams designed that in. Just as we often do when returning from the other dimensions in the dream state, I seldom recalled what I'd just spent hours preparing.

THE Guiding Light

Every day before starting the lunches or dinners I checked in with the teams on the other dimensions to find out what everyone on the programme was to eat at each meal. Often I stood and waited until I got a "hit." What resulted was frequently not at all like what I expected.

Sometimes I had no clue whatsoever about how to do a particular thing. I see now how purposeful this was. It meant I had to check "in" frequently to suss out each and every next step, one at a time. Seldom was I aware beforehand of everything that would be included. The teams however, seemed to know exactly what was in the cupboards or fridge that was perfect. I came to just trust that, as I watched my hands reach out for things which my brain found totally surprising.

In this way I can now also see how I was slowly and carefully trained to listen "up" and then follow spirit in every now moment for only the very next step, not two or three steps further down the line. This is the new paradigm for everyone. As far as tapping into the cosmic mind field is concerned, ways for doing so are shared throughout this book.

At a certain point the words oxygen therapy kept coming into my mind. I then "found" Elizabeth Baker's book *"The UnMedical Miracle - Oxygen"* and bought several bottles of 3% hydrogen peroxide and a small bottle of 35% food grade hydrogen peroxide. Zon and I experimented with the 3% on our bodies to find out what worked best for each of us. The 35% scared me away from using it at first. Then one day I just began experimenting with a few drops in our drinking water. Soon after, one person began oxygen therapy in earnest. The exact number of drops per gallon for her were designated. Her peak dose was 11 times more than what we were directed to use.

Many interesting things transpired over that time of superoxygenation. Among them, both she and I had extremely powerful, detailed and memorable dreams of other dimensional realities. I can share with you that night after night I found myself lecturing to large groups. If you attended any of these, you may recall the recurrent theme :

> It's no longer what you like or don't like or even what
> you want or don't want, that matters.

> What does matter now is that you do whatever is required of
> you to assist your human body to transform into light body.

Spirit and Humanness Merge : The Divine Human Emerges

In order for spirit, or our spiritual essence, to become one with the human body and its motive force, we need to fine tune our new focus. This is how we can tune in and turn on to what we detect through our **feelings** is spirit's direction or guidance. This may well start as a trial and error sort of thing. We can certainly tell you from our own experiences that quite rapidly we found we could pass through all sorts of trials without error as a result. This is **The Way**, the guiding light, we feel, for the coming new times. *"I have a dream..."* said Martin Luther King. It's time to live that dream.

Emerging into Light Body :
The Body of Evidence

Going Where No Human Has Gone Before : Some Signs and Symptoms

As the light body comes more and more to integrate the human body into itself, old ways of being, old ways of being simply human, fall away as we, new beings of light, take shape. Old habits, old ways of seeing, thinking, doing and being gradually, although not always seamlessly, must fall away. Some of these may be simply what and how or why you eat. Some of these old ways may also be your job, relationship, home, family, friends, resources or the kind of work you do. In whatever way best for you, spirit is speaking to you. It's saying *"Let's go get some new stuff that fits our new life together and leave all that old stuff behind."*

My observations all lead to this inevitable conclusion :

That whole new life we always wanted **has** arrived.
We simply have to unwrap it.

Breaking the Mold

From our perspective, the InterGalactic Café food programme together with the InterGalactic Clinic Therapeutics exist to simply show how new results are achieved. This is not at all through expectations or familiar formulas. After all, if you always do the same old, same old, you can only get the same old, same old. No. This is a mold-breaking process. These are mold-breaking times. You see, it's not about my plan or your plan but THE plan. And the only way to find out about that plan is by being open and honoring each step of the way "it" wants to lead you. Where you end up IS the next stage of your brand new life and the brand new you.

More Than Meets the Eye

The external changes we went through are abundantly evident. Zon-O-Ray and I both lost about 30 pounds each in about 3 to 4 months. This happened naturally, without even trying. Weekly and then daily we could feel we were not the same as we were the week or the day before as the process accelerated. It wasn't all roses. There were plenty of things to work through. There were physical, mental and emotional ups and downs. From these we gained incredible inner strengths and spiritual sustenance. We feel different, both within ourselves and to others, since this 4 month intensive began. The changes organically unfold a step at a time and minute to minute. Like breathing, you hardly notice them. It's only in looking back that we can measure how far we've come in so short a time.

Everyone on the programme noticed the differences the food was making. Their unprompted responses and reports became numerous enough to create the section called simply Some Thoughts and Feelings People Spontaneously Shared.

Like everything else in this book, we suggest you check it out to see what works for you. The real proof is when you are witness to your own changes, as joy and that incredible lightness of being seat within You.

Let Yourself Go

Health, feeling and looking good are, to me, the by-products of this forward movement into light body. This master blueprint of perfection holds the data for the perfect human beingness, the divine human. As we absorb its higher frequencies more and more into our cells, we gradually shed the human condition as we've known it up to now. We also shed the human conditioned reflexes and start to flex our light body muscles, so to speak.

This is not a time of emergency. This is an emergence. All the signs and symptoms of seeming break down whatever they may be, are the real signs of this break through. So what if you feel and act and are a little – or even a lot! – like a pubescent light being along the way. Who cares? We're not going to take any of this world with us – not even the memories. So we suggest you go ahead and let it all hang out, let yourself go. When we get to the other side, it's gonna be a whole new ball game guys. And you know what? You're part of the dream team.

Nobody said it would be a totally comfy ride. But one thing is for sure. You're not alone. Millions and millions of us are going through this equivalent of light body puberty. And it may help you to know this. You're not wacko or flaky, even if it seems like it. So go ahead, be as wacko or as flaky as you feel like. Nobody's going to remember a thing! Thank God!

What IS happening is that we are all breaking through to look and feel the new part we are about to play, taking our rightful places as cosmic citizens of new universes. It's beyond your wildest dreams. You might just like to stop in at the InterGalactic Café and Clinic to set you up on your way.

Blessings on Your journey home!

The Body of Evidence :
Some Thoughts and Feelings People Spontaneously Shared

• One night lying in bed looking at the stars, for the first time in my whole life I could feel all this space and openness inside of me, if that makes any sense to you.

• After the second or third day it felt like layers and layers, all kinds of layers, just came off. The space around me cleared. My mind got much clearer and I just feel really really wonderful.

• I can just feel the food talking to my body. I never knew I could feel so good!

• This food makes me high! I have so much energy I don't know what to do with it. After your dinner I worked for hours in my garden until it was so dark I couldn't see a thing. It was Friday night and usually I'm pretty exhausted and this was after only 3 days. I could hardly believe it. I phoned my mother to tell her all about it. Do you know what she said? She said, *"You'll never be the same again."* And I know it!

• My body absolutely craves it and I just can't eat anything else.

• I've cleared my fridge out and made this space available just for the gift of this food. Thank you for what you're doing.

• I have so much energy I'm now getting up at 5:30 or 6. I've never done that before. I'm calmer and more relaxed and seem to need a lot less sleep. I don't get angry and upset now the way I used to.

• I'm flying. Wow! I would never have believed it was possible. What did you put in there today? Can you teach me how to do that?

• Let's bottle this stuff! We could make millions. I'm high and it's legal!

• Can you fax this food to me when I get home to LA?

• I used to eat like this all the time 15 years ago. Now I'm making it for myself at home again. I can really feel the difference after eating the lunches. If the others want to eat that junk they like, they can make it themselves. Now I'm going jogging - just me and my dog at 6 in the morning.

• *Everybody said or thought on looking into the box for the first time, some variation on this :*
Gosh, that's not nearly enough. I eat like a horse and that's hardly an appetizer.

After eating, the comments went something like this :
I was really surprised. It was just the right amount. I feel full and I'm satisfied without being stuffed. I was really surprised. You know, I feel so light!

• Ok. I've decided since I feel so good eating this way that if you're not doing the food at week ends now, I'll just fast until Monday.

• I've never missed a meal in my life. I just love carbohydrates. So it was a bit surprising the other day when I didn't want to eat the baked potato with my lobster at my client dinner. In fact, I didn't even want to look at it. I just put it on a plate and pushed it to the other end of the table. A short time later I went on a fast, just naturally. I didn't know I was going to do that! I always thought fasting was OK for others but there's no way I'm going to miss my food. Three whole days! I can't believe I did that! I do feel different though. A lot different. Why is that?

• I've been chewing more thoroughly like you suggested. And really, I always thought it was a bit boring to chew. But boy, I have absolutely NO indigestion anymore. None. It's amazing. I took hydrochloric acid pills for ages. Also, have a look at my legs. I've had all these purple scars on my left leg for about 16 years. They're actually fading. Do you think that's the oxygen or the food or what? By the way, my period pains are so much better. I'm not knocked out for a day or two anymore. I feel the dragging a bit but it doesn't drain me so I have to lie down for a day like I used to.

• I've been drinking coffee for 35 years or more. I never wanted to stop and I never thought I would. I just love coffee. The other day I made this beautiful new coffee for myself and was so looking forward to it. I'd been out all day and hadn't eaten and I was really looking forward to having this coffee and being able to finally relax and be at home. After I made it when I smelled it I thought *"Yuk - I can't drink that"* and threw the whole thing away. I tried it again because I thought something must be wrong with the pot. Although I keep it clean, I really scrubbed it and rinsed it a lot. I made another potful. Same thing. Then I got it - no more coffee! It's amazing. But it's OK with me now.

I just wanted to share this with you too. I mean I just cleared out all my furniture. Stuff I could never bear to part with that belonged to my grandmother. I took it to New York and then paid a lot to have it moved out here. Well it's gone to auction in Flagstaff. All my paintings. Everything. I even cleaned out my closet and would you believe, my kitchen. It all went to "Goodwill." I threw bags and bags of stuff away. I was going to do a garage sale and I thought, why bother. I just want it out of here now. So, you know what? I've got a tent and I'm going up to Colorado. There's this meadow I saw last year and I just know I have to be there on the 23rd. I'm not sure if I'm coming back. I'll send you a post card. Lots of love. Bye.

• Every time I open the box, even after all these weeks, the smells are intoxicating. It even looks so wonderful too. I really think you've truly brought a little bit of Heaven to Earth and I thank you for the privilege of eating it and what you've done for me. I'm in Heaven.

• I never wanted to be here or in my body you know, my whole life. This is the first time I ever felt "in my body." And you know what? I actually like being here. I like being in my body. It's such a wonderful feeling for me. For the first time, really, the first time, I honor and love how my body supports me. I could never do that before. It's a wonder my body lasted me this long.

• This may sound funny. I mean it's not the sort of thing to discuss at dinner, but I really notice how my body odor has changed. I mean, I don't have body odor anymore. Here I am outside in this heat (105° plus) and my body smells sweeter, not a smelly real body smell like before. Do you know what I mean? It's really interesting.

• When we did our first cooking lesson together I took so much personally. I definitely got to see how my emotions get the better of me and how that runs around with me. Two hours spent with you was almost two hours too much. Today we've been together for what, 6 or 7 hours now and I can see how different I am and how different it all was today for me and I can see how magnificent your work is and your integrity and your truth is, even though I know I'm only just beginning to grasp it. It knocks me out. It's incredible. I love you billions.

• That tea is wonderful. It just seems to smoothen out all the lumps and bumps I come home from work with. I call it my tension tamer. I love to have some in the evening before I go to bed. I sleep so well now. We left LA after the last quake and up to now every little sound would wake me up. Now at last I feel relaxed and it's so wonderful to sleep.

• I am so excited because I see this is something I can do. My body is just buzzing. I can see how I can now work with my physical body and my consciousness. But really, I'm just so excited and enthusiastic that this is something I can **do.** It's not just words.

• I just can't get over what a difference this has made to my life. Before I was just too tired to even make a decision. Now I'm full of pep. Did you see my garden? I put all those rocks in there myself, four at a time in the wheelbarrow. If you ever want a written testimonial, just let me know.

Here is the substance of a wonderful, eye opening conversation.
It was a phone call from Miami which came just a day to two after
the food programme ended in Sedona and it simply speaks for itself.

I wanted to ask you something. I'm feeling really sick, migraine, diarrhea, gastric upset, the whole nine yards. I think it's the salad I ate. Yesterday, out of the blue, I just knew I had to eat a salad. I don't know why. I think the last salad I ate was 20 years ago. I don't like salad and I never eat it. Anyway what happened was I went to a health food store. I've never even been in one. There's a big health food store here and you'd just love it. It's got everything you can imagine. All kinds of stuff. And I just got that I had to go there.

Anyway I'm going down the aisles and I'm thinking, *"I don't know what to buy. I don't even know what I'm doing in here anyway."* Anyway so I'm looking at the stuff on the shelves and things and then I'm thinking, *"Well . . . what would zho buy? "She knows about this stuff. I sure don't."* So I start picking up stuff and asking, *"Would zho buy this? No."* So I put it back. Then I see something else that sorta flashes at me and I pick that up. *"Would zho buy this? Yes."* And I put it in my basket. So I go through the whole store like this, because I don't know anything about this stuff you know, but you know.

Anyway I get home and I make this salad. After I eat it, I'm sick. I'm talking really sick. Nausea, migraine, stomach burbling, gas – all day and most of the night. That was yesterday. Today I feel a bit better. The headache's gone. I took some pain killer. But I don't feel right somehow. I mean, what do you think?

I said that what I saw was how wonderfully she'd followed her spirit. I told her about the dream I'd had and how it's no longer about what's comfortable, or what we like or don't like or want or don't want or whatever. It's about what is required of us. Time is collapsing. Everything's accelerating. So what's required of us is how best to assist ourselves in the most graceful way possible to transmute at this accelerated rate. And how she'd just followed every step that her spirit had led her to without her brain having one single iota of an idea about what it was all about. And that she'd done this from a totally different place without questioning and rationalizing it all. Spirit was most definitely speaking to her and, like me, she was now listening "up" and doing whatever had to be done, no matter what.

I also shared with her that although it wasn't comfortable or the nicest thing in the world to have to do, we both knew exactly what it was like since we'd been through it so many times ourselves. It's a cleansing. Shit is being shifted, literally, so light can anchor in those vacated places in the cells. The light body is switching on. It's not entirely comfortable but she'd done exactly what was required. What's more, she'd done it on faith. She had gone inward and followed that implicitly. To us, that's the mark of a sovereign master in operation. And I felt that if she had ever wanted a really good example of what following spirit was, this was definitely it.

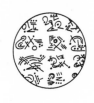

Wow, *she said.* I'm just blown away. I feel so good. I feel terrific. I feel so terrific that I almost don't notice how awful I feel at all. I mean it's there, but it's like it's no longer important. I don't have to focus on that. I see what you're saying and I'm just totally blown away by what's happened to me. As I was listening to you explaining it, I felt my focus shifted and that every word you were saying was true. It's like I knew it as soon as each word came out of your mouth. And I felt myself go yes, yes, yes. And now I can see it, it all makes total sense. I'm just blown away – So, it's that simple, huh?!

There was a short pause while she let it all sink in. Then she said – So what can I do now to really get this thing movin'? You know, I really want to go for this thing now.

Well, now I can say, There's this book you might like to read that'll tell you all about it . . .

Thanks a bunch to all concerned!

○

We are the tsunami,
the tidal wave of
the future.

Look out worlds –
Here we come !

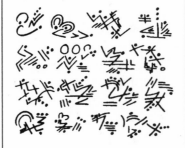

●

Doing Breakfast, Lunch and Dinner at the InterGalactic Café

△

Observing, using and catalyzing the body's three daily cycles to enhance the care and feeding of the human light body emergence.

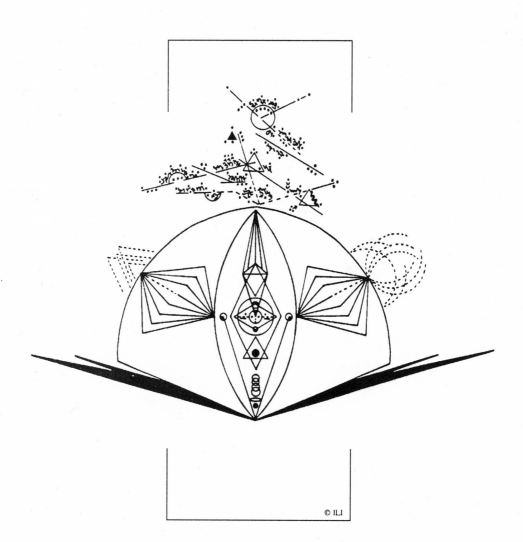

Breakfast
Organic raw fruit and/or fruit juice only

Fruit Assists the Elimination Cycle : 4 am to 12 Noon

We call the start of our day breakfast. Actually in the body's three 8 hour daily cycles it is the last of these, the elimination cycle. To assist that elimination, raw organic fruit and/or fruit juice is taken.

Fruit is a very high water content food – 80 to 90 percent water. Fruit digests in the intestines, not the stomach, in about 20 minutes. You can eat as much as you feel like up until noon, as long as it's raw and eaten only with other fruits. Cooked fruit or processed fruit juices are strong acids and toxic. Well chewed fruit needs practically no other digestion. The intestines can absorb and create energy from it rather than using energy. Whenever fruit is eaten on an empty stomach it facilitates weight loss and accelerates mutation. You return to your perfect etheric blueprint. The brain uses only glucose to function. Fruit is glucose laden brain food.

Fruit should not be eaten after other foods as in traditional desserts. It can be eaten before other foods if 20 to 30 minutes elapse first. It can be eaten after other properly combined foods if 3 to 4 hours have elapsed. It is best eaten alone and not combined with anything other than other fruit. When mixed with other foods in the stomach, the fruit rots, any protein present putrefies and any carbohydrate ferments. Everything becomes acid.

Eaten raw and alone, fruits like their counterpart vegetables at lunch and dinner, neutralize and remove hyperacid and toxic conditions built up in the body. All raw fruit and/or salad days accelerate cleansing and clearing.

Bananas and dates take about an hour to digest. Melons, so high in water content, are best eaten alone.

The cleansing action of fruit eliminates impacted deposits of grunge from the intestines. You may experience diarrhea, burping or farting. This is a good sign. Mucous membranes may discharge their toxic catarrhal grunge too. This also is good and not to be interfered with or stopped. It's all part and parcel of all the transmutative, good processes these days. It's what's absolutely right about what's happening within you. It's a process of shedding material density. And, like we mentioned before, this is an emergence, not an emergency.

In addition, like all other such regenerative, self-correcting, normal body skills and abilities, although causing temporary discomforts during mutational miracles, this too will pass.

Fruit

◦ All fruit becomes alkaline in the body and neutralizes acidity ◦

• Acid and sub-acid fruits combine well together •

blackberries	plums (sour)	apple	huckleberries
grapefruit	pomegranate	apricot	kiwi
kumquat	raspberries	blueberries	nectarine
lemon *	strawberries	cherirnoya	papaya
lime *	tangerines	cherries	peach
orange	tangeloes	fresh figs	pear
pineapple		grapes (red)	plums (sweet)

* lemons and limes are the richest food source of minerals and vitamins

• Sweet Fruit is best eaten after other fruit •

dates – allow one hour to digest
bananas – allow one hour to digest
dried fruit – allow one hour to digest
Thompson and Muscat grapes (white)
persimmon

• Melons are best eaten all alone or before other fruit •

cantaloupe
casaba
christmas melon
crenshaw melon
honey dew
musk
persian
sharlyn
watermelon

• Almonds are botanically a fruit •

And almond milk is a wonderful way to start the day.
See the "Drinks and Drinking" section for more details.

Cosmic Contact

Cosmic energy is now contacting your light body via the medium of the water in your human body. This energy is structured in a new pattern. Structured living water is a medium for this cosmic repatterning of your human body so it can mutate into light body form. Your body is 80% water and water is about 88% oxygen.

Organic Foods Carry the Highest Proportion of Life Force

Fruit assists this repatterning process since it is 80 to 90 percent water. This structured living water in fruit and other high water content living foods carries the highest proportion of the new patterns of life into your body. Organic foods evolve electron spin to photonic speeds. These evolutionary energies lead to rejuvenation and regeneration and ultimately a whole new you. You actually feel lighter as the cosmos literally beams you up .

Non-Organic Foods Run Interference in Your Field

Chemicalized foods devolve the electron spin rates. These devolutionary energies overstress the body leading to fatigue, dis-ease and degeneration. These are some of the elements the body may be working overtime to remove in order to reconnect your hotline to Heaven:

> *trace elements of 2, 4-Xylenolor2, 4-Dimenthylophenol, 6-Benzyl-aminopurine, Amitrole, AzinphosMethyl, Benomyl, Bentazon, Captan, Carbaryl, Chinomethionat, Clofentezine, Copper Sulphate, Cypermethrin, Deltamethrin, Diazinon, Dichlone, Dicofol, Dimethoate, Diphenylamine, Diquat, Dodine, Endosulfan, Etherfon, Ethion, Ethoxyquin, Fenbutatin Oxide, Fenitrothion, Fenvalerate, Ferbam, Fluazifop-Butyl, Fluazifop-P-Butyl, Folpet, Fommetanate Hydrochloride, Gibberellic Acid, Glyphosate (present as isopropylamine salt), Lime Sulphur or Calcium Polysulphide, Linuron, M-Cresol, Malathion, Manoozeb, Metaldehyde, Memidathion, Methomyl, Methoxychlor, Metriram, Metribuzin, Mineral Oil, Naphthaleneacetimide, Napropamide, OPhenylphenol, Oxamyl, Oxy-demeton-Methyl, Parrafin Base Mineral Oil, Paraquat, Parathion, Permethrin, Phosalone, Phosmet, Pirimicarb, Propargite, Propyzamide, Bimazine plus related active trizines, Streptomycin, Sulphur, Terbicil, Thiabendazole, Thiophanate-Methyl, Thiram, Methyl Bromide.*

Lunch and Dinner
Intake Cycle : Noon to 8 PM

Devolution

Chemically grown, non-organic foods may have their life force reduced by 25% to as much as 90%. Cooking them further destroys between 30% to 85% or more of what remains. The body knows what life force is. It needs it to live. It seeks it. And it will search through heaps of quantity seeking the essential life force **quality** it needs. It cannot be fooled by substitutes.

The stomach normally holds about 2 to 3 cupfuls of food. If you overeat in search of life force quality and satisfaction which just isn't there, you overload your body with dead or mostly dead foods. Dead stuff just doesn't generate life. The body becomes overtaxed, de-energized, and then gradually slows down as gobs of sludge build up. Then the big 3 D's set in, disease, degeneration and death.

Evolution

As you will notice from the lunch and dinner menus which follow, raw salads generally comprise the first part of most meals. These are high water content foods which are also alive. They are more easily and quickly digested and are eaten before the heavier and/or cooked foods which may follow. I have no data to share with you about the cooked food on the programme except to say that I did as directed. Perhaps it made things feel less regimented and more familiar and therefore more acceptable to everyone. It certainly seemed to.

The water in organic foods carries life force and information into our cells. Structurally and energetically our bodies are assisted to integrate the higher cosmic frequencies they carry nowadays. These frequencies are releasing the present human matrix. They also unlock pre-encoded data in the DNA for the human light body to come on line.

Through Kirlian photography we are enabled to see this life force in action. The auric field is pumped with light, color and movement. The electrons spin faster and faster around the nucleus of each molecule. When a certain spin rate is achieved, they expand and become photons, or particles of light. This is how we gradually, photonically, become light.

Raw organic salads, sprouts and vegetables assist us in our photonic journey.

Subatomically the force IS truly with you.

Going for a Photonic Spin
to the New InterGalactic You

Re – Evolution

When you do breakfast, lunch and dinner with the Life Force, something incredible happens :

> food addictions, coffee, tea, chemical, sugar and
> substance addictions fall away

> what's more, addictions to fear, anger, depression, victimization, inadequacy,
> powerlessness etc. diminish to eventually
> fall right out of your consciousness

The by-products of this activity are these :

> You look good. You feel good. You are good.

In a nutshell, the karmic cocoon opens and the divine human emerges.

From our perspective, when you deal with the power of subtle cosmic life forces, less of who and what you are **not** drops off and more of who and what you **truly** are results.

> Voilà. You exit the old Karma Café
> and dance right on into
> the new intergalactic YOU.

> **You wanna dance?**

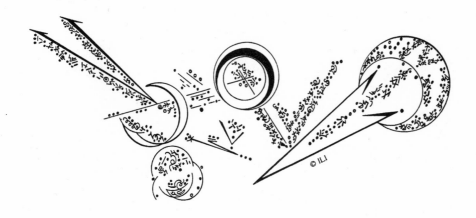

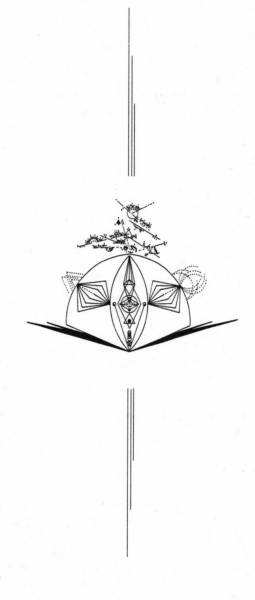

Menu
Selections
for Uncloaking

**Sixteen
chosen
favorites**

o

**Uncloaking
on the Catwalk
of Creation**

o

**Feeding Your
Energy Field
and the New
InterGalactic
YOU**

o

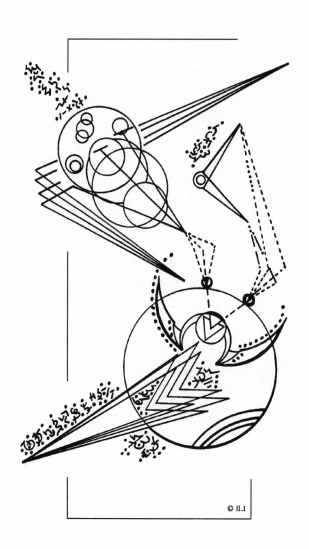

Uncloaking on the Catwalk of Creation

In order to facilitate your already entrained movement into light body, you need to uncloak.

Toxic residue, dis-ease and myriads of other discomforts with names too numerous to mention have been necessary cloaking devices. The human body is itself, a grandly designed and distinguished cloaking device. It's purpose was to dress us for the occasion thus far.

Now we're stepping into the new species look. To do that we need to first uncloak. In the aptly titled movie "Cocoon," you get a sneak preview of what your light body looks like and what it can do, thanks to special FX. No one actually has theirs yet, but, at least we know what we're going for.

This is not the end of humanity but the end of humanity as we've known it.

The new divine human steps stage center and out onto the catwalk for the whole of creation to see.

Feeding Your Energy Field
and the New InterGalactic YOU

Introduction

What follows are some tasty light infusion or light transfusion techniques. They may look just like ordinary old menus and recipes to you. Be assured, they're not. They work, or rather allow the play of subtle cosmic forces with the atomic and subatomic levels of your being. In fact, the frequencies of your bio-electromagnetic field can be altered by simply allowing your open mind to be infused and suffused by reading this book. Whether you ever do the recipes or not is another thing.

> Openness of body and mind to spirit is a new technique
> or "technology of consciousness."
> All closed systems are now opening.
> This allows new forces in to play.

Similarly the accompanying 6th dimensional light infusion transmissions brought through by Zon-O-Ray will also assist. Structurally and energetically the entire contents of this book all feed your energy field. It's just a bit of interdimensional code-talking interplay really.

On behalf of our teams and ourselves we would like to take this opportunity to say this to each member of the new species now emerging :

> You got yourself here, and you stayed,
> no matter how distressing and difficult.

> We honor you deeply and we thank you much.

It may be helpful for you to know this too. No genetic, physical, mental or emotional handicap, dis-ease or challenge will prevent your transfiguration from happening. Nothing you have ever said, done, thought or felt can stand in your way. No matter how much you've ever or never worked on your "stuff", it won't make a blind bit of difference. You are coded to do this. The codes are seeded in your DNA. You seeded yourself here and nothing and no one can stop this evolutionary upward spiral into light body.

> So the moment we've all been waiting ages for IS here.

> You were born to ascend and return to the Source.

> All the systems are now firing up.

> And, it's going to be a blast.

> •

A Word About Uncloaking and The Electromagnetic Field Effects

On the following pages you will find sixteen Menus. These were the most often mentioned "favorites" chosen by most people out of the many, many meals served.

These Menus present you with numerous ideas, suggestions and guidelines. They help build Lightworkers' intuition and inner knowing, both of which have largely been educated out of us all. Few modern manuals exist. This is one of them.

The kitchen may seem a surprising "schoolroom" to you. But it has two wonderful advantages - everybody has one and the living things which pass through its doors, such as the organic foods you will be eating, transmit force fields of communication to each and every person who desires to receive them. In addition, you can start immediately. Organic foods carry life force. This life force pulses directly into your life field or auric field, the etheric body enfolding and sustaining your physical body. You simply open both your palm chakras (pages 115 and 116) to feel it and touch it.

Organic foods taste better, too. So there is an amazing taste sensation awaiting you. Since organic foods are, in fact, the only true vehicles or carriers of life force, prana, or chi, once you get a taste for this light essence, you will notice a growing quality of light developing within your body. You just feel lighter.

A by-product of this lightness of being is that your intuition and inner knowing, or gnosis, grow too, becoming more apparent to you. You, in turn, grow to trust and stabilize yourself around this inner knowing. Inner knowing is accessed through the heart center, not the head, thus aligning the head and heart chakras in a fully operational way.

We all need a place to start once we are standing in our "schoolroom kitchen" and the following Menus form the starting points. Don't worry if you cannot find all the ingredients listed, especially those for salads. Feel free to add, subtract or substitute what may be available in your neighborhood. With regard to the recipes, however, in the Recipes for Uncloaking section following these Menus, follow them closely to fully savor their taste sensations and their alchemical formulations.

In Eastern traditions, yoga means "union with God." It doesn't apply simply to exercises or body postures but to any activity. Many people feel a sort of "greediness" in connection with food. At last we can understand the higher meaning, that we are indeed greedily yearning for that light energy which only organic or light infused foods can provide. For they enable body and soul to at last rest, in union with God.

Thus, this book could be called the *Yoga of Food* and the **Menus** and **Recipes for Uncloaking** are your exercises and homework.

Enjoy!

○ Menu Selection For Uncloaking ○

1

○ French Green Bean Salad ○

with slivered red onions, red and yellow bell peppers
marinated in a French basil vinaigrette
page 56

○ Carrot Salad ○

Finely grated carrots in an almond mayo with
fresh ginger, parsley and basil
page 57

○ Kashmiri Curry ○

Cabbage, onion, carrot, potato and celery in a
Kashmiri style curry with coconut, petit pois and plenty of hot
fresh ginger. Topped with a sprinkling of sunflower,
pumpkin and sesame seeds
page 72

○ Saffron Rice ○

Basmati and wild rice cooked in butter and vegetable stock
with all the flavors of the East - turmeric, whole black and
yellow mustard seeds, cumin and coriander seeds and cloves
and finished with a drizzle of butter
page 64

○ Cucumber Raita ○

Cucumber and tofu blended with nori and cumin seeds, fresh
cilantro and lemon, helps to cool the ginger-hot curry.
Topped with finely diced red bell pepper
page 76

•

Menu Selection For Uncloaking

2

◦ Chlorophyll Salad ◦

Finely sliced celery stalks and leaves, sprouted green peas,
young green courgettes (zucchini), grated broccoli
and finely sliced lettuce ribbons
in a garlic and basil almond mayo

page 57

◦ French Green Beans ◦

Green beans finely sliced on the diagonal with
slivered onions in a French vinaigrette
with fresh ginger and garlic

page 56

◦ The Beet Goes On ◦

Finely shredded raw beets with lots of fresh parsley and
cilantro (coriander) spiked with fresh ginger and garlic
in a French vinaigrette. Mounded on a little lettuce leaf

page 56

◦ Carrot Salad ◦

Finely grated carrots in an almond mayo with fresh cilantro,
parsley and nori flakes, sprinkled with dulse

page 57

◦ Artichoke Pasta ◦

Artichoke flour pasta has a very special flavor. The lemon butter
and basil sauce with fresh parsley and dulse accentuates it

page 60

•

• Cosmic Vibration Salad •

Finely shredded white cabbage and finely grated carrots
with plenty of fresh cilantro (coriander) and sprouted
green peas with finely sliced celery and diced sweet yellow onion
in an almond mayo spiked with extra lemon and garlic.
Nestled in a bed of lettuce ribbons and topped
with finely chopped red bell pepper

page 57

• Sechuan Tofu •

Small cubes of tofu stir fried in a hot blend
of tamari and sechuan sauces until dry and pungent.
Served on a bed of . . .

page 67

• Piquant Ginger Rice •

White basmati contrasted with shiny black wild rice.
Cooked in vegetable stock with coriander seeds
and bay leaf. Finished with a mixture of fresh ginger and mirin,
a sweet Japanese rice wine, then sprinkled
with finely sliced young green onions

page 65

• Steamed Broccoli Florets •
with a Piquant Ginger Miso Sauce

A delicious favorite
page 62

• Lemon Pudding •

A creamy uncooked tofu pudding simply
flavored with fresh lemon and maple syrup
page 91

•

○ Menu Selection For Uncloaking ○

4

• Transformational Update Salad •
Tomato and avocado wedges, cucumber cubes, celery and chopped red and
green bell peppers combine with sunflower and green pea sprouts, crisp
sweet jicama cubes and slivered Greek olives on a bed of lettuce ribbons
in a French vinaigrette with Greek oregano,
served on a lettuce leaf
page 56

• Potato-Onion Gratiné •
Thinly sliced potatoes fanned in petals in alternating
layers with thinly sliced sweet yellow onions.
Slowly simmered for several hours until the
seasonings, vegetable stock and fresh butter
are fully absorbed and the dish browns.
Served in a wedge sprinkled with
fresh parsley and cilantro
and garnished with a
black Greek
olive
page
78

•

• Life Force Salad •

Chlorophyll cranks up cellular frequencies and delivers oxygen into your body.
Thinly sliced celery, steamed chard ribbons and chopped chard stems,
lettuce ribbons, alfalfa, clover and sunflower sprouts with sprouted aduki,
mung and garbanzo beans in an almond mayo spiked with dulse,
lemon, garlic, basil and fresh ginger.
Topped with poppy seeds and Hungarian paprika
page 57

• Orange Glow Carrot Salad •

With lots of fresh parsley, dulse, cracked coriander
seeds and sweet sun-dried Greek currants
page 57

• Onion Bhagia •

A "Hindu Burger" made with potato and sweetened with
onion, finely shredded carrots and celery for crunch,
then curry spiced in hot Delhi style
served with mango chutney
page 74

• Fresh Parsley Sprigs •

When chewed to the state of liquid chlorophyll,
parsley freshens the mouth
and cleanses the palate

•

○ Menu Selection For Uncloaking ○

6

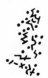

• Chloro, Phyll and Little Sprouts •

A salad of thinly sliced celery stalks and leaves, shredded
green courgettes (zucchini), with lots of tasty green
sunflower sprouts together with aduki and mung bean sprouts
and lettuce ribbons in a ginger vinaigrette with basil.
Nestled in a red romaine lettuce leaf

page 56

• Toasted Pizzaz •

A toasted pizza bun liberally spread with basil almond mayo.
Thick tomato slices, thin cucumber slices, bell pepper strips and lots
of chopped fresh cilantro are then sprinkled with lemon pepper,
Spike and dulse. The whole sandwich is then wrapped in a
large romaine lettuce leaf to catch all the yummyness

page 57

• Maple Molasses Biscuit •

A soft and moist melt-in-your-mouth biscuit
made with molasses,
maple syrup
and tofu

page 91

•

○ Menu Selection For Uncloaking ○

7

○ Green Goddess Salad ○

Romaine and curly lettuce leaves are torn into pieces and added to sunflower
and green pea sprouts, slivered green beans and green onions.
The almond mayo has dried comfrey leaf, oregano and kelp powder.
Topped with cilantro sprigs and diced red bell pepper.

page 57

○ A Walk on the Wild Side Rice ○

A fragrant, colorful and tasty mix of basmati and wild rice which is
cooked in vegetable stock and butter, colored yellow with tumeric
and larded with bright fresh green petit pois, diced red and
green bell peppers, chopped spinach and crisp celery

page 64

○ A Little Bit of Heaven on Earth ○

Chocolate pecan brownies.
No eggs, no milk, no cholesterol!
Made with tofu, maple syrup
and locally grown pecans

page 92

•

○ Menu Selection For Uncloaking ○

8

• A Green Tune-Up Salad •
A mixed green salad of sunflower sprouts, shredded broccoli,
tomato wedges, avocado and cucumber with torn lettuce
leaves in a ginger almond mayo served on
a lettuce leaf and sprinkled overall
with dulse
page 57

• Rajastani Dal •
Red lentils and onions cooked in vegetable stock and butter,
puréed and seasoned with Eastern spices (page 71) and
topped with lots of fresh cilantro
page 75

• Coconut Chutney •
Carrots and coconut are puréed and then cracked cumin
and coriander seeds are added along with dulse,
a dash of cayenne and fresh cilantro
page 76

• Saffron Coconut Rice •
Half a beautiful orange bell pepper with its green stem in place
is filled with saffron coconut rice and then
topped with fresh cilantro sprigs
page 65

• Mrs. Gandhi's Balls •
A greatly loved sweet in India
and also of the former Indian Prime Minister.
Made with garbanzo (chick pea) flour,
butter, maple syrup and pecans
then rolled in coconut
page 93

•

○ Menu Selection For Uncloaking ○

9

• Cosmic Restructuring Salad •
Celery, shredded courgettes, sesame seed sprouts, sunflower sprouts,
grated carrots, lettuce and parsley in an olive oil and
lemon dressing with garlic and black pepper
sprinkled with fresh cilantro
page 56

• Middle Eastern Falafels •
Raw sprouted garbanzos (chick peas) with raw
sesame tahini, parsley, onions and lemon are formed
into small balls, pressed and fried in tiny patties.
Presented in a lettuce leaf with a lemon sesame dipping sauce,
high in assimilable calcium
page 70

• Parsley Sprigs for Breath Freshening •

• Coconut Pecan Wedges •
A tasty, moist, chewy and filling sweet treat.
A little goes a long way
page 94

•

○ Menu Selection For Uncloaking ○
10

• Oriental "Slaw" •
Chinese leaves (napa cabbage), slivered red onion,
shredded carrot, parsley, celery and cilantro in a
ginger almond mayo with cumin seeds and
black and yellow whole mustard seeds
dusted with Hungarian paprika
page 57

• A Small Bunch of Sunflower Sprouts •
with cucumber slices
sprinkled with dulse

• Oven Roasted Potato Slices •
Brushed with olive oil, seasoned with crushed garlic and
sprinkled liberally with Spike and Lemon Pepper
presented in half a chinese cabbage leaf
page 78

• Chocolate Brownie with Pecans and Cashews •
A moist, heavenly brownie – frozen and creamy –
a sensation not to be missed
page 92

•

• Oriental Ginger Miso Salad •

Red and green romaine lettuce ribbons, sprouted soy and aduki beans,
shredded carrot with celery and parsley in an oriental dressing
– almond mayo with ginger, sesame tahini, miso and tamari –
sprinkled with fresh green onions and cilantro

page 57

• Vegetarian Sushi •

Bright yellow rice contrasts with the shiny dark green nori rolls which are
sliced on the diagonal and laid on a baby bok choy leaf.
The center of the roll is filled with shredded carrot
and celery root, baby spinach, tofu strips and
ginger miso sauce.
Radish garnish.
Fish and rice sushi are hard to digest.
Not so for vegetable sushi

page 69

• Rising Sun Salad •

Finely grated carrots in a ginger almond mayo with crushed coriander
and cumin seeds and dusted with dulse.
Accompanied by a shiny black sesame rice cracker.

page 57

• Hot Wasabi Chips •

Japanese horseradish is called wasabi. It gives zing to
your tastebuds and a buzz to your sinuses

•

○ Menu Selection For Uncloaking ○

12

• Angels In Deep Cover Salad •
An assortment of green sprouts with finely grated carrots,
parsley, celery and romaine lettuce ribbons
in a sesame tahini dressing.
Wrapped in a baby red romaine lettuce leaf
and nestled in a bed of lettuce ribbons
page 59

• Tofu Satay •
Stir fried tofu cubes in a spicy
ginger coconut sauce with broccoli florets
and fresh cilantro
page 68

• Saffron Basmati Rice •
Bright yellow basmati rice with lots of green petit pois
and black mustard seeds.
Served on a bed of steamed chard ribbons and
topped with cilantro sprigs and diced red bell pepper
page 64

• Black Sesame Rice Crackers •

•

• Enzyme Energy Salad •

Sprouted green lentils, sesame seed sprouts, chinese cabbage sprouts,
sunflower sprouts, celery, green onions, finely diced sweet red onion, lettuce,
parsley and cilantro in a French basil vinaigrette spiked with fresh ginger and dill.
Served in half a beautiful yellow bell pepper

page 56

• Tofu Cottage Cheese •

A no cholesterol dairy alternative
with dill and chives

page 68

• Tomato Slices •

Served on a bed of lettuce ribbons,
garnished with golden courgette slices
and drizzled with vinaigrette

•

*Sprouts are the powerhouse of a meal.
They are among the most concentrated
natural sources of vitamins, minerals,
enzymes and proteins on this planet.
Being biogenetic, they transfer the
streams of life force energy straight into
your body. This high quality requires
little quantity to be effective in
rejuvenation and regeneration of cells
while detoxing them too. Most
importantly of all, they carry
evolutionary resonance. The lemons
used in the vinaigrette are the richest
source of vitamins and minerals of all
and also assist detox.*

○ Menu Selection For Uncloaking ○

14

• Cosmos ComboSalad •
Lettuce, celery, parsley, jicama, cilantro, sunflower
sprouts with avocado and tomato wedges
in a basil vinaigrette with slivered black Greek olives
page 56

• Baba Ghanoush •
A Middle Eastern aubergine (eggplant) and tahini
dip served southwest style with toasted
blue corn tortilla quarters
page 77

• Indian Rice Pudding •
Raw unpasteurized milk is cooked slowly
with constant stirring until it is reduced
to a thick, golden cream.
Simply fab!

•

○ Menu Selection For Uncloaking ○
15

• Body of Light Salad •
A high water content salad of celery, cilantro, cucumber cubes,
lettuce, tomato wedges and jicama
with slivered black olives in a basil vinaigrette.
Nestled in lettuce leaves with a carrot salad garnish

page 56

• Tarragon Chicken Salad •
Shredded barbecued chicken combines with celery, cilantro,
and yellow bell pepper in an almond mayo with plenty of
spicy mustard and dried tarragon for zing.
A real taste treat

page 58

•

○ Menu Selection For Uncloaking ○
16

• The Light of Ancient Greece Revisited •
A Greek island-style salad.
Tofu cubes pressed and marinated for 24 hours replace the cheese while tasting
just like goat's milk feta. Tomato wedges, plenty of shiny black Greek olives,
thinly sliced red onions, steamed green beans, cucumber cubes,
chunks of red and yellow bell pepper and torn lettuce leaves
are dressed in an olive oil and lemon vinaigrette
zinging with Greek oregano.
Served in a lettuce leaf
page 68

•

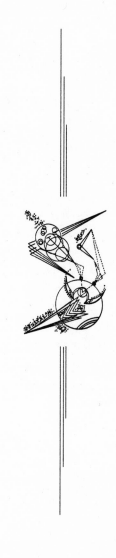

Recipes
For
Uncloaking

o

Compose

o

Consider

o

Entrain

and

Go

o

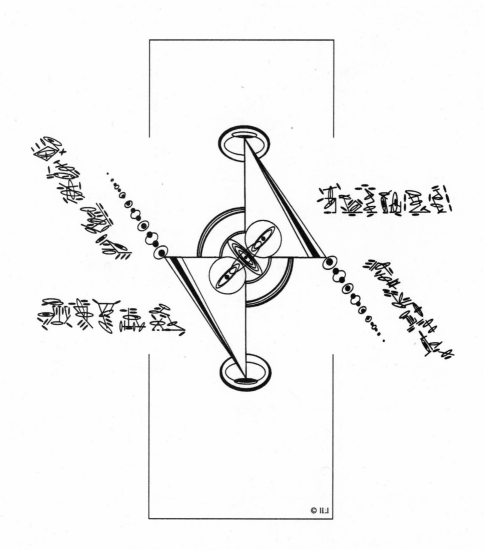

Recipes for Uncloaking
Compose, Consider, Entrain and Go

The kitchen or the dining table are fun places to play with the intelligences and forces of light. It brings in a whole new 5th dimensional meaning to playing with your food.

You can open or close the door, energetically speaking, on what you let yourself play with through the technique or technology of allowing or disallowing. The word allow, like blessing and benediction, derives from a Latin root meaning to praise. We praise things to the skies. What's going on in the skies these days? Portents and signs galore. You have friends in high places there too, and you can get higher with a little help from these friends.

So, whenever you enter your kitchen to prepare food and sit down to eat it, here are three helpful hints :

com-pose : **place** yourself **with** these friends of yours
con-sider : be **with** these **sidereal** or starry parts
entrain   : **go with this whole new flow**

These are focus techniques for the major training in listening up. Things will just naturally look up after that.

When we engage with trust in this way, our true e-ducation begins, drawing out that which already exists within.

> Each and every being is key in the
> kingdom of Heaven.

∘ **American and Metric Measures** ∘

- In this and the following recipe sections, the standard American measuring cup is used for both liquid and dry measures unless otherwise specified.
- To convert to the metric system, 1 oz equals 30 ml approximately and should be measured in a metric measuring cup.

•

French Vinaigrette Salad Dressing

6 or 7 cloves of garlic
3 level tbsp Gulden's Spicy Brown Mustard
3 tbsp raw honey
9 tbsp Bragg unfiltered cider vinegar
3/4 of a cup of a half safflower and half olive oil mixture

Press the garlic straight into your container. Add the mustard and honey mixing them well together with a fork. Then mix in the vinegar (or lemon) and then the oil so that the vinaigrette emulsifies and no oil floats.

Variations :

Cider vinaigrette is so tasty, it really needs no salt or pepper. You can ring the changes on it though, by adding to suit your palate any one of the following :

- dried basil or chives or oregano
- poppy seeds and a tablespoon of extra honey
- fresh or dried parsley and/or cilantro (coriander)
- finely sliced green onion or finely chopped red onion

Lemon Vinaigrette

Add 10 tbsp freshly squeezed lemon juice instead of the cider vinegar.

Lemon vinaigrette has a softer taste and requests the company of Spike and black pepper. Vegit or dulse and Dr. Bronner's Mineral Seasoning are possible options too.

In addition, you can add any one of the following variations :

- crushed coriander and cumin seeds, yellow or black mustard seeds and a dash of cayenne pepper
- freshly grated ginger
- a heaping teaspoon or more of sesame tahini
- dried mint and/or dill
- fresh or dried parsley and/or cilantro

The life force synergies of raw salads fill you with the energies of light and love. You can **positively** feel the difference it makes, even as you eat.

○ Both lemon and cider vinaigrette keep for about 2 weeks in the fridge in an airtight container.

Almond Mayonnaise

1 cup of whole raw almonds with their skins on
4 or 5 cloves of garlic
1/2 cup purified water (not oxygenated water)
juice of 2 lemons
1/2 to 3/4 cup safflower oil
Spike, black pepper, Lemon Pepper and a dash of cayenne
fresh or dried parsley

Almond mayo enzymatically assists brain mutation.

Grind the almonds finely in a seed mill or blender.
Add the garlic, water and lemon juice and blend all together.
Add the oil and blend until smooth.
If it's too thick, add a little more water and/or lemon juice.
Add the herbs and seasonings to taste.

Carrot Salad

Finely grate as many carrots as you need, 4 to 5 say, using a Japanese grater for very very fine shreds. Add enough basic almond mayo to ensure that the salad is well mixed with the mayo without being soggy or mushy. Add lots and lots of fresh parsley.

Serving Suggestions :

You can ring the changes on carrot salad by adding the following variations :

- Menu 1   add enough freshly grated ginger for a sharpish gingery taste and some dried basil
- Menu 2   add fresh cilantro (coriander) and nori flakes and then sprinkle the servings with dulse or Hungarian paprika
- Menu 3   add dulse, cracked coriander seeds and a few Greek sun–dried black currants
- Menu 11   add dulse, cracked coriander and cumin seeds and freshly grated ginger

○   Carrot salad keeps for a week or so in the fridge in an airtight container. If you have made a lot, use it up by garnishing other salads or dishes with its lovely orange glow.

Menu 15 : Chicken Salad

Take enough mayo for your finely shredded chicken salad and add a tablespoon or two of dried tarragon and 2 to 3 tablespoons of Gulden's Spicy Brown Mustard to taste. Add 20 to 30 cracked coriander seeds which give little bursts of taste when you chew them and perhaps a little freshly milled black pepper, Spike and Lemon Pepper. You could also add cajun spices or cayenne if you like a bit of a hot kick. Some finely sliced celery stalks and leaves give chicken salad some crunch and fresh cilantro gives a lovely taste sensation. Add your finely shredded chicken and serve the salad dusted with Hungarian paprika.

- You can crack or crush whole coriander seeds by pressing them with the back of a teaspoon in a small bowl.

Variations on Almond Mayonnaise :

From your basic almond mayo remove sufficient for the salad variation you want to try out, put it in another container, and then add any one of the following to suit your palate :

- lots of freshly grated ginger
- a couple of teaspoons of Gulden's Spicy Brown Mustard. This is great with celery, parsley and onions for potato salad.
- a couple of teaspoons of tahini, extra lemon, mint and/or chives or sliced green onions
- extra fresh and/or dried parsley and/or cilantro (coriander)
- cumin and/or coriander seeds crushed
- poppy seeds or dried dill or oregano
- To "curry" the mayo add freshly grated ginger, crushed cumin and coriander seeds or powder, a dash of cayenne or cajun spices, black or yellow whole mustard seeds, Spike and Lemon Pepper. If you really want to be creative, also add a couple of dashes of cardamom powder and allspice or garam masala.
- You can thin the mayo to a salad dressing consistency by adding extra lemon juice (not vinegar) and olive oil to taste and perhaps a little mint. You can vary that still more by adding any of the variations above.
- Either plain, or with any of the variations above, a thick garlicy mayo also makes a great dip accompanied with crunchy raw veggies for a party treat, appetiser, or as a centerpiece of a salad plate or party buffet.

- Almond mayo keeps for a week or two in the fridge in an airtight container.

Sesame Tahini Sauce and Dressing

3 heaping tbsp raw tahini
2 to 3 cloves of garlic pressed
juice of one lemon or more
3 to 4 tbsp of olive oil
Spike, Lemon Pepper and cayenne
lots of fresh, finely chopped parsley

Mix the pressed garlic and tahini together with a fork.
Add lemon, olive oil and a little water so the dressing is thick but manageable.
Add the seasonings and parsley to taste.

Serving Suggestions :

- Sesame tahini sauce makes a good dip for raw veggies, pitta bread and falafels as well as crackers

- It makes an unusual and earthy tasting salad dressing. You can keep it thick or thin it with a little more lemon (not vinegar) and/or olive oil. Taste variations can include : mint, mint and dill, oregano, comfrey, or nori flakes.

- You might like to sprinkle the finished salad with black or white sesame seeds, pumpkin and sunflower seeds, plenty of paprika, onions, or slivered black Greek olives.

- It replaces mayo on sandwiches or burgers and can be added as a swirl on soups, or to thicken sauces.

Sesame seeds are a wonder food and together with almonds
are a high calcium dairy replacement.

○ Sesame Tahini Sauce keeps for weeks in the fridge in an airtight container.

Butter Sauces : Brain Mutation Food

Butter is a real fat, and neutral. Vedic tradition holds clarified butter or ghee to be brain food and is a much valued liquid gold. What makes cows holy is their horns which transfer and transduce cosmic energy into their bodies to be passed on in the liquid called milk.

We use *"Alta Dena"* butter and organic ghee which are not adulterated by man-made bovine growth hormone (rBGH). A butter sauce occasionally on fish or vegetables is a taste treat. However, since cooked tomato is highly acidic, butter's greatest use is as a sauce for pasta.

Incidentally, acidic conditions actually leach the body's calcium to neutralize them. We can get more than adequate calcium from raw, organic nuts, seeds, fruits, green leafy vegetables and dates. The cow gets its calcium from chloro and phyll in grass and from seeds. For humans, raw sesame seeds have the highest most assimilable calcium content of all.

Butter Sauce for Pasta

14 to 16 tbsp butter or ghee
3 or 4 bay leaves , several cloves of garlic
basil, Spike, black pepper, Dr. B's minerals, cayenne

For each 3/4 pound or so of raw artichoke pasta which you have cooked, melt about 14 to 16 tbsp of butter in a heavy stainless pan or pot. This prevents the butter from browning or burning. Turn the heat to low and press several cloves of garlic into the melting butter and add all of the above herbs and spices to taste.

Simmer on low for about 10 to 20 minutes covered. The sauce thickens and changes consistency but the butter should definitely not brown. When done, add to the cooked pasta and stir the sauce in well.

Here are some tasty variations :

- use a half butter and half olive oil mix
- oregano can be used instead of basil
- try some freshly grated ginger (p. 61)
- Lemon Butter Sauce, or a lemon and olive oil sauce, or a sauce using olive oil instead of butter are other alternatives to ring the changes if you're a pasta lover. Pasta and cheese are a real digestive no-no. Pasta and cooked tomato sauce are too.
- Fresh tomato salsa makes a wonderful and instant pasta sauce.

Some additional serving suggestions :

- All of the butter sauces are great with vegetables, vegetables and rice, or steamed vegetables with a good bread to dip up the sauce. Yum yum.

- The cooking water from the artichoke pasta can be used when cooled, to nourish ailing outdoor plants or to feed healthy ones

- Keep one bottle of olive oil with several peeled and slivered garlic cloves to flavor the oil and to save time. You can also add a hot chili or two if you like it hot. This also doubles up as a very occasional appetizer treat for dipping foccacio bread into.

*On a number of occasions our lunch boxes came back squeaky clean. When we said to people "You know, you don't have to wash the boxes, just close them and we'll wash them when they come back" their answer was "I didn't wash it". Just how they licked these boxes clean was a mystery to us. But it did cause us to let you know that because the food actually **works**, burping and farting – all within reason, of course – are all quite natural at the InterGalactic Café, along with licking your plate.*

Lemon Butter Sauce for Fish

4 to 6 tbsp butter	1 or 2 tsp dried dill
2 or 3 bay leaves	3 to 6 tbsp lemon juice
Spike, Lemon Pepper, black pepper, Vegit, dulse, kelp	

I cover raw fish fillets with a slightly diluted 3% hydrogen peroxide and purified water solution for 10 to 15 minutes in a glass container. This detoxes it before cooking. Then melt 4 to 6 tbsp of butter for each pound or so of fish on medium heat in a heavy stainless pan with a close fitting lid. Poach the fish gently on both sides. The butter should not be allowed to brown. Remove the fish to a plate when it's about half cooked. Add all the other ingredients except the lemon to the sauce. Cover and simmer on low for another 5 minutes. Turn up the heat and add the fish juices from the plate and the lemon juice and stir. Then cover and turn off the heat for several minutes. Now add the fish, warm the pan on low for 3 or 4 minutes or until the thickest part of the fish is translucently white, not raw looking and also not "dead" white and overcooked. Serve immediately.

- You can freeze partially cooked fish portions plus sauce in cling film for another time. You can then nuke the thawed portions for a minute or so prior to serving for a quick meal .

Piquant Ginger Miso Sauce

Mix together to a thick consistency :

3 tbsp mellow white miso

2 tbsp raw honey

2 tbsp raw sesame tahini

3 tbsp rice vinegar or lemon juice

1 tbsp grated fresh ginger

a few drops of water if needed

Serving suggestions :

- This is a lovely sauce on rice. Because it is so concentrated, you need only a coffee spoonful per portion of rice or vegetables.

- Very very slightly thinned, it's wonderful on hot or cold veggies.

- It will add zing to your vegetable sushi rolls.

- It's amazing with raw carrots as a dip, or mixed into steamed julienned carrots with a drop of two of carrot steaming water.

- It livens up plain slices of broiled or pan fried tofu or plain stir fried tofu cubes.

- It works as a salad dressing for high water content celery, cucumber cubes, cilantro, bell peppers and sprouts.

- If it becomes too thin and runny, add a touch of almond mayo to thicken it up and a touch of tamari to lift the taste.

- Piquant Ginger Miso sauce keeps for weeks in the fridge in an airtight container.

Basic Vegetable Stock

All garlic and onion peels and other bits of unused vegetables which are usually cut off and discarded can now go into a large tupperware in the freezer. Mine is a 48 fluid ounce size. Carrot ends, cilantro and parsley stalks, the tough outer celery stalks, courgette ends, broccoli stalk peelings, potato eyes (I don't peel root vegetables), green onion roots, fennel fronds, etc etc. Each time the lidded container fills up, I put all the contents in a pot, cover with about 3 cups of purified water and simmer it for 45 minutes to an hour after it's reached a boil. Leave it for about 24 hours and strain.

- What makes this stockmaking process so interesting is that it is so varied. The vegetable pieces you may have collected at one time may not resemble those from any other times. You can add a bay leaf or two if you like and bits of onion if you haven't enough peels. Red onion gives the stock a bright red appearance and garlic sharpens the taste.

- I put 1 and 1/2 cups of the vegetable stock into one pound plastic tofu containers and freeze the container in a plastic bag. This makes measuring for rice simple, since 1 and 1/2 cups of stock are required for each cup of raw rice to be cooked.

- Stock is also useful to have on hand for a miso soup base or bean or lentil soup base or for potato gratiné or for whenever else vegetable stock is needed for a quick rice or soup dish.

- If you steam your vegetables in very little water, you can collect that in tofu containers too. Or you can feed plants with it. It's best to use this nutrient laden liquid in a life enhancing way.

Basic Chicken Stock

All the chicken bones, skin etc can put into a lidded pot and covered with 2 to 3 cups of purified water with a bay leaf added. Simmer it for about an hour, covered, on the lowest setting after it has reached a boil. After it cools, leave it overnight in the fridge. Warm the pot to melt the jelly and pour off the stock through a sieve. It's very very tasty as a soup stock.

If you prefer a concentrated stock, use about 1 and 1/2 cups of water.

I freeze chicken stock in one cup covered containers for quick meals.

- Here's a delicious and instant pick me up. To a cup of hot chicken stock, add a teaspoon of vegetable or wild mushroom concentrate such as *The Organic Gourmet* brand. With a rice cracker and butter or warmed pitta or toasted Indian Meal bread, it's fast and rich, filling and heavenly. What more could one want? Enjoy!

Basic Saffron Rice

1 and 1/2 cups of vegetable stock (15 oz)
1 cup of basmati rice and a handful of wild rice (11 oz)
turmeric, bay leaves, coriander seeds and cumin seeds
yellow and black mustard seeds

Method of Preparation :

This rice is a most beautiful yellow color. Tumeric colors the rice less expensively than saffron while adding its own special flavor. This is further enhanced by the aromatic addition of cumin and coriander seeds as well as mustard seeds.

Basmati rice looks and tastes elegant when combined with a small handful of beautiful shiny black wild rice to contrast with the yellow.

I usually make only one cup of rice at a time using a 10 oz glass coffee cup as my measure. When the 15 oz of stock boils in a heavy bottomed stainless pot, add the wild rice first, cover and allow it to boil for 3 to 4 minutes since it takes a little longer to cook. Then add a heaping 1/2 teaspoon of tumeric, a bay leaf or two, 20 to 30 whole coriander seeds, a couple of pinches of cumin seeds and a quarter teaspoon of yellow or black mustard seeds.

Cloves are an option you may like to try sometime as is a dash of nutmeg, or cinnamon, or allspice, or 5 or 6 cardamom pods cracked to release their fragrance.

Add the 1 cup (10 oz) of basmati, allow the stock to come back to a boil, stir to distribute the rice evenly in the stock and replace the lid. Lower the heat to the lowest setting and time for 20 minutes. Do not remove the lid during this time. Turn off the heat and allow the rice to rest in the still unopened pot for about 5 minutes more on the burner.

Move the rice to a cool burner, remove the lid and gently fluff the rice with a fork. Replace the lid until you're ready to serve.

Rice should only be cooked in a heavy pot so it does not burn or dry out. It also will stay hot for about 10 minutes or so and warm for about half an hour.

Your whole kitchen will be aromatic and fragrant with the smells which will definitely stimulate your whole body not to mention salivation.

- This recipe is for standard white basmati rice. If you can obtain organic white basmati, it requires about 22 minutes to cook. Vedic basmati rice imported from India and Pakistan continues to be harvested by hand as it has been for centuries. Standard commercial processing practices such as bleaching, oiling, pearling and powder-coating diminish both flavor and nutritional value. This is no way to treat this lady, this queen of ancient grains.

Menu 3 : Piquant Ginger Rice

Add the white Basmati rice to boiling stock or water, plus 2 to 3 bay leaves, 6 to 8 whole peppercorns and a teaspoon each of cumin and coriander seeds. When cooked, fluff the rice with a fork while gently stirring in a mixture of 2 tbsp mirin (sweet Japanese rice wine) or 1 tbsp honey, 3 tbsp brown rice vinegar and a little freshly grated ginger to taste. Basmati is a delicate rice and mushes if you are not gentle with it while it's hot. Cover the pot and let the flavors meld for 5 minutes or more.

Serve the rice garnished with finely sliced green onions or fresh coriander or topped with a coffee spoonful of Piquant Ginger Miso Sauce.

Menu 8 : Saffron Coconut Rice

Add a tablespoon or two of butter or ghee for each cup of raw rice you've used and stir it gently through the basic saffron rice. Then add a small handful of shredded dried coconut, spritz it with some oxygenated water and stir it throughout the cooked rice too. Cover and let it stand for 5 minutes or more before serving.

Alternatively, add the coconut and the butter to the stock with the raw rice prior to cooking along with an extra tablespoon or two of stock or water.

Serve the rice topped with fresh cilantro or parsley sprigs.

A Few Serving Suggestions :

*   Any rice takes on a party look when served in half a beautiful bell pepper of any color.
*   Add frozen petit pois after fork fluffing the rice. The peas heat up while retaining their beautiful bright green color and most importantly, their taste.
*   You can add finely shredded carrots as well as, or instead of coconut while fluffing the rice with butter. A few dried black currants makes this an appealing, extra special dish.
*   Hot saffron rice or coconut saffron rice topped with a little butter and a sprinkling of dulse granules, nori flakes or black sesame seeds is a colorful and simple taste treat on its own
*   Cold rice can be reheated by steaming briefly. Add julienned carrots, broccoli florets, petit pois or any leftover veg you may have on hand. Steam everything together for about 2 minutes.
*   If you prefer to nuke your rice to reheat it, spritz with oxygenated drinking water first and cover the glass container loosely.
*   A tasty alternative to butter is to top each portion of rice with a small coffee spoonful of Piquant Ginger Miso Sauce and then sprinkle that overall with finely chopped green onions or cilantro or chives.

Tofu

Tofu is a wonder food to assist light body emergence. Made from soybeans, it is not only cholesterol free, it actually lowers existing blood cholesterol. It's a high water content food. This makes it an extremely light and digestible protein. Its alkalinity also neutralizes existing acidity in the body. Half a pound of tofu contains about 50% of your daily protein requirement and up to 43% of usable calcium. This is more calcium than in milk and eggs yet tofu is far more easily digested and absorbed than these animal products. Tofu also contains essential omega-3 fatty acids without the cholesterol burden of fish oils, as well as lecithin which helps dissolve fat in the body.

It is a wonder food in other ways too. Tofu can taste just like meat. Especially after being frozen, it has a chewy, meat-like texture. It can taste like cottage cheese, feta cheese or cheese cake. It can taste like milk and eggs in baking and substitute for them. It transforms and transfigures itself. In the new human paradigm of wholeness, this ancient food of the East finally and fully contacts the cellular mind of the West.

Preparing Tofu :

One pound blocks of organic tofu are available in your health food store for about $1.50 or so. Remove it from the container and cut off the amount you need if you're not using it all. Squeeze the block gently and then cut it into even slices crosswise. Lay the slices flat on paper towels on a cutting board and cover them with more kitchen towels. Add another cutting board on top. As a weight I use 2 full gallon containers of drinking water. The objective is to press as much water as we can out of the tofu prior to using it. All tofu is usually prepared in this way whether it is cooked or to be used raw.

Pressing
The longer tofu is weighted down, the better it is for cubing. The average time I leave if for is an hour or two. But 10 to 20 minutes is OK if you're in a hurry.

Storing
Any tofu you are not using should be stored in an airtight container in the fridge, submerged in fresh purified water which is changed every other day. The original water from the package should not be re-used for this. Do check the date stamp before buying your tofu to ensure that it is as fresh as possible.

Reviving
Slightly stale tofu can be revived by being submerged in a stainless steel pot of boiled purified water. Let it sit for a few minutes covered. This can then be used at the time or frozen for another time. Fresh tofu can be frozen too.

Freezing

To freeze tofu, I remove it from its container and gently squeeze the water from the block taking care not to crumble the edges. After feeding the plants with the liquid, replace the tofu block in the container. Then the tofu plus container goes into a plastic produce bag and into the freezer.

When you are ready to use it and it has thawed, cut, wrap and press the tofu as outlined above. Frozen tofu makes the best cubes because the consistency becomes spongy after freezing. This absorbs and holds a lot of the yummy sauce we're going to use for Sechuan tofu. But freezing is not absolutely necessary. Sechuan Tofu is very forgiving. No matter what you do, it tastes wonderful.

Cubing

Don't worry about the size of the cubes you'll be cutting. If you've not worked with tofu before, don't worry. Even if your block crumbles, this recipe still works. I like to make 1/4 inch slices, stack them after pressing and cut 1/4 inch strips lengthwise and then 1/4 inch crosswise cuts. This gives you lots of 1/4 inch cubes. It's something you may or may not aim for. Do what works for you. Size and shape don't really matter. What matters is the enjoyment it gives you in doing it and then eating it.

- The water in the plastic tofu container is an excellent food for plants. I dilute it with a bit of tap water. A small dying magnolia tree revived and bloomed within weeks when fed three times a week.
- The plastic tofu containers are stackable and make for excellent flat storage of vegetable or chicken stock in the freezer.

Menu 3 : Sechuan Tofu

The recipe couldn't be simpler. For a pound of tofu cubes I use about 7 tablespoons of tamari and one or two tablespoons of Sechuan sauce. Add more hot sauce if you like a fiery taste. Mix together in a bowl with a fork.

Stir fry the cubes in a hot wok with a little safflower oil for about 2 to 3 minutes on high heat, add the sauce and stir fry until the cubes are dry. Remove the wok from the heat and let the cubes cool, or use them immediately. Voilà. Sechuan Tofu par excellence. Like we said, it couldn't be simpler.

Serve Sechuan Tofu on a bed of rice or mounded in a lettuce leaf. Hot or cold, it tastes excellent.

- Add Sechuan Tofu cubes to salad for a hot and spicy zing.
- Mix Sechuan cubes, rice and frozen peas and nuke for a 40 second meal.
- Add the cubes to miso soup or mix them with steamed carrots, broccoli or any vegetable you want to enliven. You can also use them in, or to accompany, sushi rolls.
- Sechuan Tofu cubes can be rolled in lettuce leaves with rice and/or vegetables for a fun food presentation.

Menu 12 : Tofu Satay

Take about half a cup of dried shredded coconut and pour over one cup of hot, not boiling water. Cover and let it stand for a few minutes. Then blend the mixture for a minute or so until it's creamy. Combine this in a saucepan with one envelope of "A Taste of Thai Peanut Sauce Mix" (mild or medium) and simmer together for 5 or 6 minutes until it thickens up. Add a pound of crumbled or cubed tofu and simmer it in the sauce for about 10 minutes or so.

- Just before serving, pass your left hand over the pot and invoke the force of light to vitalize the dish for the highest good of all concerned. Feel the vibrations rise to meet your hand so you know when this is completed. I use this technique to vitalize anything which is questionable.

Serve the Tofu Satay on or with rice and sprinkle the portions with finely sliced green onion and fresh cilantro.

Menu 13 : Tofu Cottage Cheese

I cut a pound of tofu into 4 or 6 parts and squeeze them as dry as I can by hand. Crumble about half the tofu into a container and keep the rest aside. Add a tablespoon or two of safflower oil, 2 to 3 tablespoons of lemon juice, 2 to 3 tablespoons of nutritional yeast, Spike, Lemon Pepper, dulse, kelp, Dr. Bronner's Minerals and a dash of cayenne or cajun spices. Blend to a cream. Then add one or two green onions finely chopped, a tablespoon or more of freeze dried or fresh chives, a tablespoon of dried dill and a teaspoon or two of cumin seeds and mix them together with a fork. Then mash in with the fork the tofu you had set aside so the tofu has a lumpy appearance and the texture is like that of dairy cottage cheese.

- An alternative is to add a tablespoon or two of cider vinegar with the lemon juice which gives a spikier taste.
- You can also add a little chopped and seeded hothouse cucumber.
- Still another variation is to add oregano or basil instead of the cumin seeds along with some grated black pepper.
- I like to present it sprinkled with paprika or dulse and a shiny black olive in a lettuce leaf with finely chopped red or yellow bell pepper.

Menu 16 : Greek "Feta Cheese" Salad

Frozen tofu works best if you have time, otherwise just cut, wrap and press the tofu as above and marinate the cubes in a little lemon vinaigrette for 10 to 20 minutes, or overnight for a stronger taste.

After the salad has been tossed, mix in the cubes just before serving.

- You can also mound the "feta" cubes in the center of a salad for a different feel, adding plenty of parsley, green onion and/or fresh cilantro.

Sushi

Nori is a sea vegetable, dried and pressed into greenish-black and lustrous sheets about 8 inches square. This seaweed should be toasted before using, according to the instructions on the packet. Sometimes called sushi nori, but more often just Nori, it is used to make sushi. Aonori, or green nori, is the flaked variety we use sometimes as a condiment since it is so rich in iron and protein. Rice and fish sushi are a no-no combo for digestion. Rice and vegetables on the other hand, are a good combo.

I like to use yellow saffron rice to contrast with the bright green of the toasted nori. When the rice is hot, it sticks together well. You can add the mirin, rice vinegar and freshly grated ginger as in Piquant Ginger Rice for an added and authentic oriental sharpness, if you'd like.

Have ready some of the following, or anything else that takes your fancy:

avocado   sushi ginger
cucumber strips   sunflower sprouts
finely shredded jicama   finely shredded celery root
ginger miso sauce or wasabi or umeboshi paste
lightly steamed baby spinach
tofu strips or cubes, Sechuan Tofu style
finely grated carrot and/or broccoli stems peeled and grated
finely grated radishes, or Japanese black radish or pickled daikon radish

Lay the nori flat after toasting on a bamboo nori-maki mat or a cutting board. Add a few tablespoons of rice across the nori so it is heaped up a little higher on both outer edges. Press this down with a fork to avoid it falling out when you come to roll it up. Add your choice of ingredients following the list in **Menu 11** or select from some of the ingredients above, laying them out over the rice and distributing them evenly from side to side.

Then roll the nori up as tightly as you can into a cylinder, starting from the edge nearest you and rolling away. Wet the farthest edge very slightly along its length and roll the cylinder to form a seal along that edge. Let the roll rest a moment on the sealed seam while pressing back in with a fork any rice which may have fallen out of the cylinder ends during the rolling.

Wet the knife and damp dry it clean on a wet sponge or cloth between each diagonal cut. I make 6 diagonal slices from each roll and present 3 or 4 of these sushi slices so that they overlap and either stand up or lie flat.

Sushi is definitely worth the effort to get the hang of it.

Sushi rolls do not keep well. If you do need to refrigerate them for a short time prior to serving, place them on a plate with a bowl to cover. Plastic wrap makes the rolls go soggy.

If your rolls come out tasting rather bland, don't worry. A tasty dipping sauce can be made by reconstituting wasabi powder, a green Japanese horesradish, plus a dash or two of tamari or shoyu. Wasabi has quite a kick. If you've not used it before, do a taste test with the teensiest amount first!

Hummus and Falafels

The Copts are an ancient Christian group in Egypt. They claim to be the pure representatives of the ancient Egyptians. Ta'amia is their national dish, made from dried white broad beans. But it has also become the Israeli national dish made from garbanzo beans or chick peas, which we have come to know so well as falafels. Everyone just loves them. Perhaps they trigger whispers of ancient memories of the cradle of civilization logged in our cells.

This recipe allows you to make both hummus "salad" and falafels too. Both these dishes are very forgiving and the garbanzos are earthy, simple and infinitely variable as well as almost impossible to spoil.

Method of Preparation :

Soak a pound or so of garbanzos overnight in enough water to cover them. Drain and cook them in purified water with 2 or 3 bay leaves in a heavy, covered pot for about an hour or so, until they are soft. Drain, reserving a few whole garbanzos and a small amount of cooking water. Use the remainder of the soaking and cooking water to feed your plants. They'll appreciate your thinking of them and caring about them and they'll be inordinately grateful.

For every 10 oz of cooked garbanzos use 2 heaping tbsp of raw sesame tahini and 2 pressed cloves of garlic and the juice of 1 to 1 and 1/2 lemons. Add 1/4 cup of olive oil and blend. If the hummus is too thick, add a little of the cooking water to thin it a bit. If you're going to make falafels only, leave it as thick as possible.

For Hummus

Add a little cayenne, Spike and 5 tbsp of fresh parsley and or dried cilantro for each 10 oz of cooked beans you've used. An interesting variation is to add dulse and nori flakes.

Serve dusted with sweet Hungarian paprika and a sprig of parsley along with the few whole or slightly crushed garbanzos to garnish the servings. Traditionally hummus is served with warmed or lightly toasted pitta. You may like to try raw vegetable crudités to ring a tasty change. Hummus is also wonderful heaped up on rice crackers or black sesame rice crackers or water biscuits. It's also a great dip for blue corn or other chips.

For Falafels

For each cup of hummus which we will now turn into falafels, add a couple of tbsp of chopped sweet red onion, 2 to 3 heaping tbsp of fresh parsley and enough whole wheat or pitta or other nonwhite breadcrumbs mixed with a teaspoon or so of baking powder to make a wettish mixture.

Form this into small balls and press with a fork or spatula to make patties about 1 and 1/2 to 2 inches in diameter and 1/2 an inch or so thick. Fry the falafels in safflower oil in a wok on medium high until they are brown on both sides. Let them rest on kitchen towels to absorb excess oil.

The texture of falafels should be dense so that they hold their shape well without crumbling. They also freeze well for another time. Serve the falafels with a sesame tahini dipping sauce.

Indian Cuisine : East meets West

Curry is a simple, elegant and taste filled "way" or tao of cooking and eating. Derived from an ancient living culture, it may at first seem mysterious and complex. But we can pop this illusion quite simply.

You will find bulk herbs and spices in your local health food store. For a dollar or two you can stock up with a couple of tablespoons of each of the following aromatic Eastern mysteries. Commercial curry powders bear absolutely no resemblance to the real thing which we are about to prepare.

Eastern Mysteries Revealed :

The herbs and spices listed here are basic to Indian cuisine :

whole black mustard seeds
cumin and coriander seeds
cumin and coriander powder
cardamom pods or powder
turmeric
bay leaves
cayenne pepper
whole cloves
powdered nutmeg
garam masala
fresh or ground ginger
yellow mustard seeds can be substituted if
black mustard seeds are not available

You will also need some fresh or dried parsley, fresh or dried cilantro, dried shredded coconut and some sea salt. Indian cuisine requests safflower oil. Olive oil is far too heavy for the delicate aromatics we will be working with.

With these few elements we can now unveil an eastern mystery or two.

Cabbage Curry

Almost anything can be curried. In the recipe which follows, we will prepare a cabbage curry. Cauliflower, broccoli, chicken, beef or tofu, lentils, beans etc etc can all be curried in the same way. So, let's start.

You will need a heavy largish stainless steel pot with a tight fitting lid
and the following vegetables :

3 to 4 small onions cut in half, each half cut into 8 wedges
one large 2 to 3 lb. white cabbage finely shredded
2 to 3 large carrots finely sliced on the diagonal
3 to 4 potatoes finely sliced or diced with the skins left on

Optional additions may include :

green beans
2 to 3 celery stalks and leaves
frozen green peas
fresh parsley or cilantro (coriander)
3 to 4 oz of dried shredded coconut

The herbs and spices :

1/2 tsp. black (or yellow) mustard seeds
3/4 tsp turmeric, 3 to 4 bay leaves
several pinches of cayenne pepper
1/2 a heaping tbsp each of cumin and coriander seeds
1 heaping tsp each of cumin and coriander powder
6 to 7 whole cardamom pods or 1 tsp powder
fresh ginger or ginger powder
garam masala

Method of Preparation :

Curry is about what you have and what you create out of a few simple things. So there is no standard and this recipe is only a starting point for your creations.

Heat the pot on medium high and add 3 tbsp safflower oil. When the oil is hot, add the black mustard and cumin seeds. When they sputter and pop, add the onions and the bay leaves.

Stir the onions to prevent burning and cook them until they are transparent, then turn the heat to high, and add the potatoes. While these brown, put the finely shredded cabbage briefly under cold water in a collander. With the heat on high, move the onion and potato to the edges of the pot to maximise the central area available for the cabbage you are now adding to contact the hot, browned bottom of the pot. If your pot hasn't browned, don't worry. Just carry on. Stir well.

Sprinkle on the tumeric, cumin and coriander powders, a dash of cayenne and a couple of dashes of Dr. B's Barleymalt Sweetener or a pinch or two of sugar. Add the cloves and fresh ginger if you've decided to use them and stir to distribute everything throughout the wilting cabbage.

Add the carrots and stir them in to prevent any scorching. Then with the heat still on high, add purified water to a depth of an inch or two and bring that to a boil. Add cardamom pods and coriander seeds and a sprinkle of sea salt. Stir, put on the lid and reduce the heat to medium for 10 to 15 minutes.

Check the liquid level adding more water to maintain an inch or two in depth and now stir in the cut green beans if you're using them, along with fresh or dried parsley and/or cilantro. Stir everything again, cover and reduce the heat to low for about 20 or 30 minutes or until the potato breaks down and thickens the curry. When done, the curry should be thick and chunky, with softly crisp carrots.

Just before serving add the celery, frozen peas, finely chopped bell pepper, fresh cilantro, the coconut and stir them all in thoroughly so that the flavors meld together well. Add cardamom powder now and a teaspoon of garam masala if it's available in your area. Adjust all seasonings and add more salt and cayenne to suit your palate.

I find that curry likes to rest a bit, covered, on the hot burner for a further 10 to 15 minutes before being served.

Garnish with :   * a paper thin lemon slice
                        * finely sliced green onion
                        * fresh cilantro sprigs or parsley sprigs

- The amount of curry given here is sufficient to allow some to be portion frozen for quick meal appeal another time. Some of it can then also be used for the Hindu burgers on the next page.

- Cabbage curry improves with age as the flavors meld. It keeps a week to 10 days in the fridge in an airtight container.

Hindu Burgers

Take the driest part of the curry off the top. Alternatively, drain any leftovers you have in a collander. Reserve the liquid. It can be added to soups and sauces. You can poach vegetables in it, simmering until the sauce thickens more and the vegetables are cooked. If any is still left over, use it again another time as a sauce for rice or potatoes etc or freeze it for another use. This sauce can also be thickened with mashed potato, potato flour or cornstarch for a "gravy" on other foods.

Back to the burgers :

Purée or mash the curry to a rough chunky consistency that is still smooth enough to shape into burgers. Add some whole wheat or stale pitta breadcrumbs (but not white breadcrumbs), a few mustard seeds, cumin and coriander seeds and fresh or dried parsley. The mixture should be firmish and wettish, not stiff and dry. Then shape and fry the burgers as below.

Onion Bhagia

For this variety of "burger," add some thinly sliced or finely diced raw onion, a little grated ginger and some finely shredded carrot along with the breadcrumbs or garbanzo flour to bind the mixture together.

Take enough to form flat patty shapes about 3 or 4 inches in diameter. Heat a wok on medium high, add a little safflower oil and fry 6 or 8 burgers on the bottom until brown.

Turn and brown them in a little more oil. The burgers should be about half to three-quarters of an inch thick.

Serve with *Major Grey's Mango Chutney* or *Major Grey's Bengal Hot Chutney* or cucumber raita, or a lemon wedge. They are sensational, soft and intriguingly delicious.

- A variation is to add a little mashed hard style tofu which gives a slightly harder burger.

Rajastani Dal

Lentils are inexpensive and high in protein. This dal delight is made from quick cooking red lentils and is very easy to digest.

You will need :

red lentils soaked for 10 to 15 minutes
several onions
vegetable stock or water
bay leaves and curry spices

Method of Preparation :

For each half pound of red lentils, chop 2 small onions. In a heavy stainless steel pot heat a little safflower oil, add the cumin and black mustard seeds and when they pop and sputter, add the onions. Stir on medium high heat until the onions start to brown slightly, then add the drained lentils and 2 to 3 bay leaves and stir them together briefly in the hot oil. Feed your plants with the soaking water from the lentils. They love it.

Add about 1/2 cup or so of water or stock for each 1/2 pound of lentils used. Bring the liquid to a boil and add the curry spices to taste. Stir, cover and reduce the heat to low and cook for about 20 minutes or until the lentils dissolve into a mush. Purée with a blender. The dal should be thickish like mashed potato.

Add a little sea salt and some chopped green onion or cilantro or parsley and a little garam masala and stir them in. You can also add a few cloves if you'd like to try a slightly different taste. Let the dal rest to harmonize the flavors and fragrances for about 5 to 10 minutes before serving.

Rajastani Dal can be served hot or cold with a thin lemon twist or wedge.

Dal Soup

You can make soup from this same recipe by simply adding more stock or water and spices to taste.

- Serve the soup with a thickish lemon slice floating on top and sprinkled with fresh cilantro.
- Alternatively swirl a little sesame tahini slightly beaten with lemon and a dash of safflower oil through the surface of the soup as you would do if using sour cream.
- Still another garnish is to add a dab of fresh butter to melt over the surface of the soup.

Possible Variations on Dal Soup :

Use flat green lentils, split green or yellow peas, or mung beans to give you several variations on this theme. Soak these overnight with enough water to cover. Proceed as with red lentils except for the little longer cooking time which may be required.

Curry Loves Company

Cucumber Raita

Yogurt in various forms often accompanies an Indian meal. It freshens the palate while cooling it too. Tofu is a wonderful substitute in this simple alternative dairy free version.

Take about 1/8 pound of hard style tofu and crumble it into a container with a little lemon juice, Spike, Lemon Pepper and a dash of safflower oil. Blend with a hand blender until creamy. Stir in some finely chopped cucumber, nori flakes or dried or fresh parsley, some crushed cumin and coriander seeds or powder, some fresh cilantro chopped finely and a dash of cayenne to taste.

A nice presentation is to place a spoonful or two in a small lettuce leaf or a small Japanese dipping bowl, sprinkle the raita with a little powdered cumin or cumin seeds, or paprika, or dulse granules and add paper fine slices of cucumber alongside for garnishing.

Coconut Chutney

A couple of spoonfuls of shredded dried coconut are steeped in enough warm but not boiling water to wet the coconut. Pulse the mixture with the blender until it becomes smooth. Add a couple of tablespoons of shredded carrot. If the chutney is watery, drain it in a sieve until it has a dryish texture. Cracked cumin and coriander seeds are added and a little dash of dulse along with the merest hint of cayenne and a few chopped or whole cilantro leaves.

Heap a tablespoon or two of chutney along with a cucumber slice on or alongside the curry.

Baba Ghanoush

This is a rich, creamy and earthy aubergine (eggplant) and tahini dip, sharpened by lemon and garlic according to your palate.

You will need :
1 medium or large eggplant or several small ones
3 to 4 cloves of garlic
1/4 cup raw sesame tahini
juice of 2 or 3 lemons
Spike, ground cumin and some crushed coriander seeds
lots of fresh parsley
a dash of cayenne pepper
a good pinch of cumin powder
2 to 3 tablespoons of olive oil

Wash, dry and pierce the aubergines in several places with a fork. Bake in a hot 450 degree oven. The aubergines will collapse as they become very very soft and squishy. Turn them occasionally to assist the softening process and prevent them from burning. They may need up to 1 and 1/2 hours to soften if they are large.

Remove the soft mushy flesh from the skin discarding any hard parts as well as the stem end. Mash with a fork or blender adding the rest of the ingredients to taste.

I like it sharp and earthily seductive.

Serving Suggestions :

Baba Ghanoush is great as a dip with raw vegetable crudités, or toasted pitta quarters, or warmed blue corn tortilla quarters, or blue corn chips.

You can also serve it as a centerpiece to a salad plate with a few shiny black Greek olives and dusted with paprika.

It is also a tasty dressing and garnish when generously spooned over thick tomato slices, perhaps accompanied with some cucumber slices or cubes, on a bed of lettuce ribbons.

Potato Onion Gratiné

Arrange very very thinly sliced potatoes, 1/16 inch thick with their skins on, in a half inch layer on the bottom of a large shallow casserole. Add a few rounds of paper thin onion slices over the whole of the potato surface, sprinkle on a little potato or other flour and season the layer with Spike, Lemon Pepper, freshly milled black peppr, dried parsley or basil or cilantro and a few dashes of Dr. B's Minerals or dulse granules. Then add a few thin shavings of cold butter.

Continue alternating the layers until you have three-quarters to one inch left at the top of the dish.

Pour over sufficient hot or cold stock to just barely cover the potato and add a few more shavings of cold butter and the seasonings. Should your potato slices float because they're too thick, put a plate over to weigh them down until they soften and subside.

Slowly simmer the dish at 350 degrees until the butter and stock are fully absorbed and the surface browns. This could take several hours if your casserole is large. I prefer glass so I can see when it's done. There should be no liquid left and the potato should be firm enough to cut into wedges.

Serve the gratiné hot or cold in wedges with sprigs or sprinkles of fresh parsley or cilantro and garnished with a shiny Greek olive.

Oven Roasted Potato Slices

Turn the broiler to high and while it heats, slice 3 or 4 potatoes in 1/8 inch thick slices. Combine 6 or 7 tablespoons of olive oil and 2 to 3 pressed garlic cloves in a small bowl and beat them together.

Brush the broiler pan with this mixture, arrange the potato slices on it and brush them too. Season with Spike and freshly milled black pepper. Broil the slices as close as possible to the heat, removing those which may brown quicker, until all are done.

Simple and delicious, these roasted potato slices need no dipping sauce.

To ring a change, mist the slices with fresh lemon juice after broiling and use Lemon Pepper before broiling.

Serve in an overlapping regiment in a small lettuce or tender chinese cabbage leaf.

Seasonings

The seasonings we work with are these :

Spike All Purpose Natural Seasonings (Modern Products)
Lemon Pepper Seasoning (Modern Products)
Vegit All Purpose Seasoning (Modern Products)
Dr. Bronner's Balanced Mineral Seasoning
dulse granules
kelp granules or powder
black pepper freshly ground in a pepper mill

Herbs and Spices :

dried and fresh basil	dried dill
bay leaves	oregano
coriander powder and seeds	cayenne pepper
cumin powder and seeds	Hungarian paprika
tumeric	cloves
black and yellow mustard seeds	fresh ginger root as an
garam masala	aid to digestion

For Masala Chai or Indian tea :

whole cloves
allspice
cardamom powder
cinnamon

Other Condiments :

Gulden's Spicy Brown Mustard
Bragg organic unfiltered apple cider vinegar
bulk grade B maple syrup
mellow white miso and brown rice miso
mirin, a sweet Japanese rice wine
tamari, any macrobiotic brand
raw organic sesame tahini

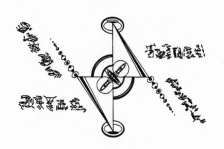

Drinks
and
Drinking

o

Chew Your Liquids
and Drink Your Foods

o

Mystical, Magical Water

o

Almond Milk

o

Coconut Milk

o

Oxygenated Water

o

Masala Chai
or
Indian Spiced Tea

o

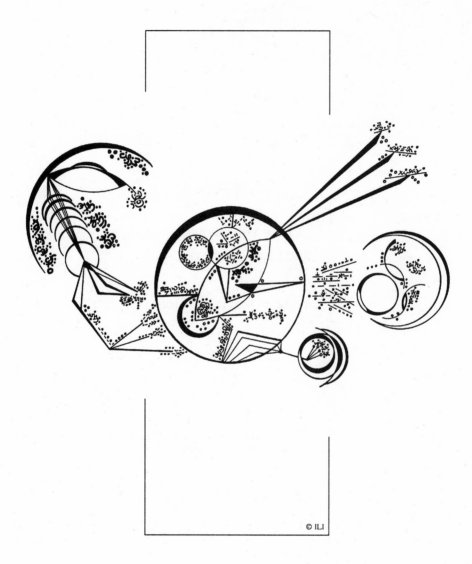

© ILI

◦ **American and Metric Measures** ◦

- In this and the following recipe section, the standard American measuring cup is used for both liquid and dry measures unless otherwise specified.
- To convert to the metric system, 1 oz equals 30 ml approximately and should be measured in a metric measuring cup.

Drinks and Drinking

Chew Your Liquids and Drink Your Food

Most people don't chew their food well and so have to wash it down with a drink. Mahatma Gandhi advises us to chew our liquids and drink our food. Why? Saliva well mixed with food starts the digestion process in the mouth and triggers the necessary gastric secretions for enhanced digestion by the stomach. Chewing well also breaks down the cell walls of raw foods and makes smaller particles and therefore less of a burden on the other digestive processes which follow. Liquids introduced other than those naturally occuring in the food, dilute the stomach's secretions. The stomach is not designed to digest lumps of unchewed food. Lumps floating around in diluted and/or neutralized liquids? ... Well, you can see the point.

To facilitate weight loss, slowly drink and "chew" a full 10 ounce (300 ml) glass of water about an hour before eating. Drink at least 60 to 80 ounces of water (1.8 to 2.4 liters) each day between meals. In connection with food, drink only about half an hour before or at least one hour after eating. Oxygenated water is good. Fruit juices, like fruit, should be fresh and raw. They can be taken about 20 minutes to half an hour before a meal but should not be taken within 3 to 4 hours after non-fruit meals.

Alcoholic, carbonated and caffeine drinks are definitely detrimental. At present, it is an astonishing fact that Americans drink more manufactured drinks than water. It is also an astonishing fact that soft drinks and our "quick fixes" of tea, coffee and alcohol require at least two 10 ounce (600 ml) glasses of pure water to neutralize them. They not only dehydrate our bodies but, more importantly, they dehydrate the brain and overload the kidneys.

On the other hand, nut milks are rich in organic nutrients. Almond milk in particular contains an enzyme which facilitates brain mutation. Fruit juices and smoothies as well as veggie juices are tasty, satisfying and assist detox. All liquids should be "chewed" thoroughly to assist the preliminary digestion by the saliva, though perhaps not for the 150 times Gandhi suggested!

On the food programme we prepared almond milk, oxygenated water, masala chai, an ayurvedic type of tea and occasionally coconut milk. People had this at tea-time around 4:30 or 5 in the afternoon, about 4 hours or so after lunch. Except for warm tea, all liquids should be drunk at room temperature. Ice and cold drinks shock the system and the body shuts down its biological processes to deal with this "red alert."

Remember, nothing is chiseled in stone. If your spirit guides you to eat a McDonald's hamburger, OD on pizza or ice cream, down a bottle of cola or a beer (the hops assist mutation) or even smoke – Follow Your Spirit.

One of the things which becomes very very apparent at some point is when you begin to discern when your spirit directs you and when your addictions do. Once you know which is what, things get very very clear, very very quickly.

Until then you might just be a puppet on a craving's string.

Mystical Magical Water

Water is a magical and mystical medium because it can be "charged" or imprinted to store subtle energies. The subtle energies which are imprinted can be either harmful or helpful. Healers, homeopathics, flowers, gems and certain symbols for example, can charge or imprint water with positive, nourishing and elevating vibration.

Angry, depressed and ill people can also transmit and imprint their negative, de-energizing and devolutionery vibrations into the high water content of our food and our drinks. Chemical farming does the same. The human body which may be exposed to such dis-ease charges, or **imprints**, requires only positive frequencies to shift upwards into health. This upward shift is called **resonance induction**. The lower or negative vibrations are called, or induced, into higher frequency octaves to resonate in harmony with health. This is also known as **evolutionary resonance** since Nature is constantly perfecting her creations through evolutionary or upward cycles. Any higher resonant frequency which the body may encounter assists it to "discharge" any toxic frequencies or lower vibrational imprinting which it may have picked up along the way. Hindrances obstructing this process create what we call a "healing crisis." Health or healing crises are good. They help us to surrender to go with the "natural flow." Mother Nature always seeks to provide for her children by moving them towards health and away from sickness.

Mudra, mantra, meditation, prayer and the laying on of hands are just some of the various ways in which we can flow with Mother Nature's natural "cure all" energies, if we give time, opportunity and conscious understanding on our part. For it is the etheric imprint or vibrational pattern of the Divine Mother which gives birth to material substance and Man, not the other way around.

> Understanding and working with this gives the baseline
> reference of energy medicine for the next millennium.

What does all this mean to YOU?

Simply that your "hands," pure plant food, pure water, natural products, intention, will and yantras or pictorialized frequency patterns (page 120) can have deeply penetrating bio-informational effects through the process of "energy transfer." These energy transfers zap dis-ease and induce health by means of higher frequency imprints. Water is the all-pervasive medium for this. Everyone possesses that inner power within themselves which can be released in service to this world as energy medicine.

About two-thirds of our planet and 99% of our cells are water, so we have indeed, a huge potential for healing and purification at our very finger tips. More about this in the following chapters.

Almond Milk

Introduction

The almond has been around for ages. Botanically a fruit, it combines well with other fruit. It is, in fact, the ancient ancestor of today's apricot, peach, plum and nectarine.

Have you noticed how much "ancient" stuff is included in this book? Perhaps the almond, like the banana and the rose, was seeded here as a help to mankind from our ancestors in another time and place in space. This is why it's important to follow your spirit rather than anything or anyone "outside." Genetically you are being called to by your ancient heritage as the light bearer of that ancient lineage.

Almonds are a complete protein source, containing all 8 of the essential amino acids. These are "essential" to the human body but are not manufactured by the human body. If you've found yourself wanting almonds in some form, raw, in cakes or sweets or whatever, your assistance is being requested in the brain's mutational sequencing.

Method of Preparation :

10 oz of almonds with their skins on
48 oz purified water
5 tbsp maple syrup

Grind the almonds to a fine meal.
Add 1 cup of water and blend until thick.
Add another cup and blend for a minute or two.
Add the remaining water and blend for several minutes.

Leave overnight in an airtight container in the fridge. Then strain the liquid through an extra fine sieve into a jug or other airtight container. Add the maple syrup and shake well to mix.

- Almonds have an enzyme not found in other foods which supports whole brain mutational functioning. Almond milk is a wonderful and soothing drink anytime and makes a delicious fruit salad accompaniment. It replaces milk and soft drinks and needs to be refrigerated.

- Almond milk keeps for 3 to 4 days in the fridge.

- **Beauty Tip:** The leftover almond meal makes a wonderful face and body scrub which leaves the skin unbelievably silky and soft after showering or bathing. It also needs to be kept in the fridge in an airtight container. It freezes well, too.

Because almonds are a fruit, almond milk makes a good breakfast treat
either on its own or added to fruit salad.

Coconut Milk

4 cups of water warmed slightly to "blood" heat
1 cup of dried shredded coconut
2 tbsp maple syrup

Blend the coconut with 2 cups of the warmed water for a minute in a blender. Strain off the milk into a jug or other container. Then pour the remaining 2 cups of water over the pulp and blend again. Strain again.

Add 2 tbsp of maple syrup to the milk in your jug and shake it well to integrate it all together. Your container should have an airtight lid.

The leftover coconut pulp can be frozen to add to soups, sauces or curries.

○ Coconut milk keeps only about 2 to 3 days in the fridge. If the cream hardens during chilling, let it stand at room temperature for a bit and then shake it vigorously to integrate the cream. It is simply delicious.

Oxygenated Water

Drinking

We add between 7 to 9 drops of 35% food grade hydrogen peroxide to each gallon of purified water.

You can add one drop directly into your glass with a dropper if you prefer. Be sure to stir it in well before drinking though.

Spritzing

We keep a plant spray bottle in the kitchen to spritz lettuce leaves, leftover salad, and cooked rice before nuking it for a meal, etc. We use a half and half mixture of 3% hydrogen peroxide and water for this.

Soaking

Any meat or supermarket produce is soaked for 2 to 3 minutes (or longer for large pieces of meat) in a glass bowl with a half and half mixture as above, or according to your own inner directions.

Making 3% Hydrogen Peroxide

We found a stainless steel one ounce (30 ml) coffee measure and we use it to add one ounce of 35% food grade peroxide to 11 or 12 ounces (350 ml) of purified or preferrably distilled water. This produces a 3% hydrogen peroxide solution which can be kept in the bathroom for body oxygenation as well as in the kitchen for spritzing and soaking commercially grown fruits and vegetables as appropriate.

35% food grade hydrogen peroxide is best refrigerated so it retains its full potency over time. Straight 35% burns your skin so do be very, very careful when handling it.

Additional information on oxygenation can be found on pages 118 to 121.

Masala Chai : Indian Spiced Tea

3 cups of purified water
3 Twinings brand Orange Pekoe Tea Bags
2 cups of raw milk
3 big pinches of cinnamon powder
4 big pinches of cardamom powder
1 big pinch of allspice
2 big pinches of freshly milled black pepper
6 to 7 whole cloves
1 tsp honey per serving

Boil the water in a heavy stainless steel pot. Turn off the heat and add the teabags. Cover and leave the tea to steep for 4 to 5 minutes.

Remove the tea bags, add the cloves, milk and then all the spices. Turn the heat to high and beat the spices in with a spoon so they are fully dissolved and integrated.

When the tea reaches a boil again and froths up, turn off the heat and strain into serving cups.

Add a teaspoon of honey to taste.

Keep any leftover tea in the fridge in an airtight container. For subsequent servings, strain into cups and nuke for a minute to a minute and a half.

This tea is something else! Most people commented that they could absolutely feel its calming and healing properties. It's major communiqué seems to be :

Everything's just fine. No worries.

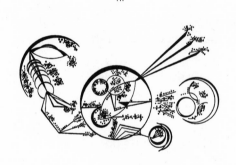

Pie
in the
Sky

o

Six
Simply
Heavenly
Sweet
Treats

o

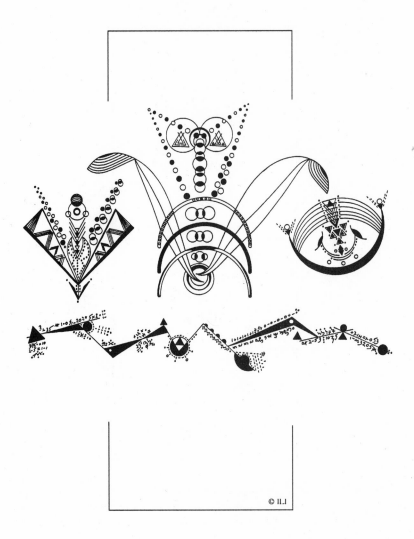

© ILI

○ American and Metric Measures ○

- In this recipe section, the standard American measuring cup is used for both liquid and dry measures unless otherwise specified.

- To convert to the metric system, 1 oz equals 30 ml approximately and should be measured in a metric measuring cup.

Lemon Pudding

Blend together until creamy :

3 to 4 tbsp safflower oil
3 to 4 oz maple syrup
a dash of sea salt
1/2 tsp vanilla
6 tbsp lemon juice
1/2 lb. hard style tofu

Chill well to set it before serving.

- Use 6 tbsp cocoa powder instead of the lemon juice for chocolate pudding.

- A variation is to add coconut shreds or pecans for an extra special treat.

Maple Molasses Biscuits

8 oz molasses
10 oz maple syrup
10 oz safflower oil
1/2 lb hard style tofu

35 oz unbleached white flour
1 tsp salt
1 heaping tsp baking powder

In a largish container, blend the first four ingredients together until creamy using a hand blender. In a separate bowl, integrate the next three ingredients together well. Then stir the dry ingredients into the tofu mixture with a spatula until the mixture is well blended and is dryish and stiffish.

Heat your oven to 350 degrees. Form balls of just under 1/8th cup of batter and place them on your oiled broiler pan or baking sheets using a spatula to press them down so that 2 or 3 ridges are formed on the surface. You will get 50 to 60 biscuits about 2 and 1/2 inches in diameter.

Bake them for about 25 to 35 minutes or until they're done. They should be soft without being gooey inside, yet not hard on the outside or dark on the bottoms.

Store the biscuits in an airtight container in the fridge and freeze a portion if you can! They're so yummy they may disappear before you have a chance.

Heavenly
Chocolate Pecan Brownies

4 oz unbleached white flour
6 oz purified water
1/2 lb. hard style tofu

20 oz maple syrup
2 tsp vanilla
8 oz cocoa powder
5 oz safflower oil

15 oz unbleached white flour
2 heaping tsp baking powder
a few pinches of sea salt

8 to 10 oz of pecans or cashews, or a combination of both

In a saucepan whip the first three ingredients together until creamy. Stir this mixture over low heat until it thickens and then cool it for 5 minutes in the freezer, not forgetting to set the timer.

Meanwhile, in a bowl combine the next 4 ingredients well together. Then add this to the tofu mixture and stir it all well together with a spatula.

In another bowl, integrate the next 3 ingredients well together with a fork. Add this to the tofu mixture. Stir until it's smooth and lump free. Then stir through the pecans or cashews or both.

Bake in two 8 inch or 9 inch stainless steel pie plates for 45 minutes to an hour at 350 degrees or until a knife inserted in the center comes out clean.

To serve, cut the cooled brownies into 8 or 16 wedges.

Store the brownies in an airtight container in the fridge or freezer.

• They make a wonderful "frozen" dessert straight from the freezer.

Mrs. Ghandi's Balls

This most popular Indian sweet was also something the late Prime Minister, Mrs. Indira Ghandi favored, purportedly, and so the name we gave it was . . .

14 tbsp butter or ghee
20 oz sifted chick pea (garbanzo) flour
measured after sifting
4 heaping tbsp dried shredded coconut
1/4 heaping tsp nutmeg
8 oz of maple syrup
6 heaping tbsp smallish pecan pieces
7 heaping tbsp dried shredded coconut, pulsed until fine

Melt the butter in a very heavy bottomed pan on medium heat. Mix the flour, nutmeg and 4 tbsp of coconut together well in a bowl and add to the butter. Stir with a wooden spoon for 3 to 4 minutes taking care the mixture does not burn by scraping the bottom and the sides of the pan constantly.

Add the syrup, continue blending, stirring and scraping the mixture for another 4 or 5 minutues on medium heat, ensuring it does not burn. Add the pecan pieces, turn off the heat and continue stirring gently for another minute or two.

Take the pot off the burner and let it rest for several minutes.

Then spread the mixture onto a glass cutting board or other surface with a spatula.

When it's cool enough to handle but still warmish, roll pieces of the dough between your palms to make 60 or 70 little balls. Then roll these into the 7 tbsp of finely shredded coconut, then between your palms, so the balls are covered with coconut.

Refrigerate in an airtight container. Some can be frozen for another time – if you get the chance! We rarely did. They're also great straight from the freezer.

Coconut Pecan Wedges

10 oz maple syrup
3 to 4 oz safflower oil
5 tbsp lemon juice
2 tsp vanilla
1/4 lb. tofu

15 oz unbleached white flour
1 tsp sea salt
5 oz roughly ground oats
10 oz dried shredded coconut
1 and 1/2 heaping tsp baking powder

8 oz of pecans or cashews or a mixture of both

Blend the first five ingredients with a hand mixer in a large bowl. In a separate bowl mix the next five ingredients together well and add them to the liquid ingredients, folding the mixture well together with a spatula. Then add the nuts.

Divide the mixture between two 8 inch diameter pans and bake at 350 degrees until a knife inserted in the center comes out cleanly, about 50 minutes or so.

Cut into 12 or 16 wedges and serve.

Store the rest in an airtight container in the fridge or freezer.

Indian Rice Pudding

Be prepared for about an hour of stirring. This recipe derives from Indian temple cooking and is very much about bringing cosmic energy down the spiral of the clockwise or figure 8 stirring motion. We use raw unpasteurized milk free of hormones, antibiotics and DNA altered materials.

3 or 4 tbsp butter or ghee
5 to 6 ounces of white basmati rice
3 bay leaves
3/4 gallon of milk (96 oz)
10 oz maple syrup
1/2 heaping tsp of cardamom powder
a small handful of sun-dried Greek currants

Melt the butter in a very heavy bottomed large stainless steel pot on medium heat. Stir–fry the rice in the butter until it's transparent, then add the bay leaves and the milk. Continue to stir on high heat with a wooden spoon until the milk froths up in a boil. This takes about 10 to 15 minutes. Take note of the milk level on the perpendicular wooden spoon before the milk boils. This dip stick measure will serve us later on.

Continue stirring on high heat for about 25 to 30 minutes more. I do my breathing exercises while I stir, as follows :

IN   through the nose to a count of 7, expanding the abdomen
HOLD to a count of 7
OUT   through the mouth to a count of 7 pressing the belly towards the spine using the diaphragm muscle
HOLD to a count of 7

Do this seven times and then intone as follows :

three OM's as follows : OHHHHHH as low as possible in the belly area for a count of 7

MMMMM nasally with the teeth clenched to vibrate the skull bones for a count of 7

Do remember to keep stirring though !

When the pudding has thickened and reduced by about 25% from the original dip stick mark you noted earlier on, add the syrup and cardamom. Continue to stir slowly but constantly to prevent scorching. After about 10 to 15 minutes you will get the feeling that the right thickness and creaminess has been obtained.

The pudding continues to thicken as it cools, so remove the pot from the burner, put on the lid and let it cool after stirring in the currants.

Refrigerate until well chilled and set. **This is truly, ambrosia from Heaven.**

- For a real "cool" treat, freeze the rice pudding in small portion containers and eat it straight from the freezer.

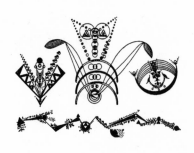

Self-Purification and Self-Healing

○

Alchemical Detox

○

Alchemical Cleansing

○

Alchemical Renewal

○

The Alchemical Formula for Food Combining

○

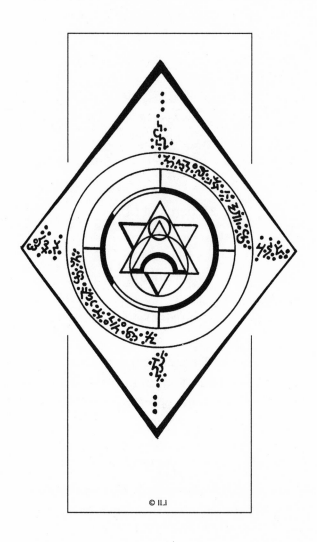

© ILJ

Self-Purification and Self-Healing

Both this chapter and the following chapters present several high profile ideas.

Firstly, it is our considered opinion that each one of us here is spirit having a human experience and therefore there is nothing which we cannot do.

Secondly, although this world has told us otherwise and few manuals exist which speak from this point of view, this is our baseline from which to build, using the various simple but effective "alchemical formulae" presented.

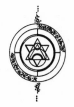

Thirdly, it is also our considered point of view that when you initiate yourself into the modern mystery school in the temple of your body, high vibrational foods are your perfect high vibrational energy medicines to do so.

This and the upcoming chapters are about evolving your necessary lifestyle changes. They present you with various ways to help you self-implement these changes, slowly but surely.

As we see it, your body is the laboratory for an experiment in Self-realization by Self-actualization. Mother Nature is the midwife and this is our virgin birth.

There is nothing which we present here which we have not tried out first on ourselves and also on a few other people besides. So it's not theory, but facts which work.

Lastly, we are making "light" of all we say and do. This is our means for working with high energy and as flow directors of Light. For laughter really is the very best energy medicine. What's more, if we can do it, so can you.

And on this note, please get ready to turn over a new leaf.

I. Salidization Provides Alchemical Detoxification

In general, lunch and dinner meals in this transformational food lifestyle begin with a high water content raw salad. Any vegetable which can be eaten raw can be saladized. We serve salad on a lettuce leaf or on a bed of lettuce "ribbons" as well as including lettuce pieces torn by hand in the salad. Its high silica or clear quartz content holds high frequency resonance in the body the same as quartz crystals do in radio receivers. Like CB radio, the human body is a transmitter receiver of Cosmic Band frequencies.

Lettuce Leaves

Lettuce leaves are carefully rinsed under cold running water and then laid out to dry, carefully arranged in absorbent hand towels. I have six pure cotton "bathroom variety" hand towels kept in a kitchen drawer for this sole purpose. You can choose any color that suits your spiritual needs of the moment. Mine are golden yellow.

If your lettuce is not organic, the leaves can then be spritzed lightly on both sides with a mixture of half purified water and half 3% hydrogen peroxide and then laid in layers in the towels.

Roll up the stack of towels tightly into a big "log" and let the leaves dry for 10 to 15 minutes or so. When the leaves are ready to use or to store, blot off any excess water which may be left in particularly curly or overlapping parts of the leaves. Any wetness, especially on tender curly lettuce or baby lettuce leaves, causes them to wilt. Water in your salad will make it waterlogged and soggy instead of crisp and light. So do ensure that your lettuce leaves are well dried.

You can wash and store enough lettuce leaves for several meals in a large and roomy airtight container which is kept in the fridge. Simply lay the well-dried leaves between layers of paper kitchen towel. They will often remain crisp and crunchy for several days if organic lettuce is stored in this manner.

In addition, you will always be able to fix a quick salad and be sitting down to eat in five minutes or less. This helps us to eat well while also coping with busy workday schedules.

Lettuce Ribbons

Lettuce ribbons are easily made by stacking several leaves together, folding the top down towards the stem end and then rolling from one curly side towards the other. You end up with a big roll like a Havana cigar which makes it easy to cut 1-1/8 inch wide ribbons without cutting your fingers.

Mixed Salads

All mixed salad elements apart from the lettuce are generally sliced or shredded finely and diced small. Such ingredients might include zucchini, shredded carrots and/or parsnips, celery, bell peppers, sprouts, beetroot, cucumber, daikon radish, fresh or thawed petit peas and so on. Tossed together, the salad presents well on the plate, and, the pieces being so delicate, offer more surface for the vegetables and the lettuce to take up the tastiness of the salad dressing. Small pieces seem to encourage people to chew more and thus savor their food more, too. People in a rush find they can slow down and this is something everyone always mentions. Good digestion can then take place normally and without digestive aids.

Organic Economies

Because organic foods are whole and packed with life force, one or two big handfuls or so of salad are adequate for a meal which is also going to be accompanied by a condensed or cooked food, whether protein, starch or vegetables (page 106). Three or more big handfuls constitute a good general serving if a main course salad is all you are eating. Raw organic salads will start to desludge your intestinal tract, provide vegetable protein and structured intelligence in the high water content of the cells, along with fibre, and should optimally form at least 50% of the weight of your lunch or dinner. Organic foods may seem expensive at first, but you eat less of them since the life force they contain charges or imprints you with health and "discharges" the vibrations of dis-ease.

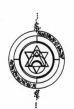

Sharp Knives

A sharp knife slices cleanly and precisely so the cells of high water content foods are not mutilated to then wilt from the rough handling of a blunt knife. My all time favorite knife and the one I use most often is a *Kershaw* with a 4 3/4 inch (12 cm) serrated blade, model 9921 in case you are interested. It's made in Japan and can be ordered by any good Knife Shop outlet. *Kershaw* also makes an excellent and lightweight cook's knife, too. The finest instruments always give the best physical and energetic results.

Alchemical Formula #1
Salads Produce Alchemical Detoxification and Self-Healing by:

• structured, intelligent water carrying subtle energies and evolutionary "codes"

• raw chlorophyll which builds blood, allowing greater cellular oxygenation

• the removal of intestinal parasites and viral/bacterial overgrowth

• raw fibre to cleanse and purify the entire digestive tract

• a new feeling of satisfaction without being "stuffed"

• a new sense of lightness and well-being

• weight loss of general toxicity

• the ability to walk more

"lightly" upon the planet
renewed with a
sense of
Grace

•

II. Olive Oil and Lemon Provide Alchemical Cleansing

Olive oil and lemon juice are the Mediterranean staples of salad making. The purest extra virgin olive oil is expeller-pressed and the premier mono-unsaturated oil. It has been prized as an energy food and an energy medicine since ancient times. In fact, olive oil is the best carrier of medicinal ozone, meaning extra oxygenation and detoxification for your system. The finest Greek olive oils have distinctive characteristics and flavor and pure Kalamata olive oil is my favorite.

No other oil can ever really replace olive oil because most other oils are refined and highly processed. The oil is separated from its food source by the use of petroleum solvents. These cheap oils are then refined at high temperatures with highly toxic solvents and chemicals. After refining they are bleached and deodorized and lack not only aroma and flavor, but vital nutrients and oxygen, too.

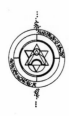

Although simple, olive oil and lemon juice are quick and easy, tasty salad dressing ingredients requiring no preparation, especially if you've run out of vinaigrette. Just drizzle the oil and lemon over the salad, add Spike and black or cayenne pepper, toss and eat. And these ingredients can be elevated to their highest states, as in the ancient mystery schools, via your cosmic consciousness infusion. They become the very ingredients of sacred initiation, handed down the eons from Atlantis, through Egypt and then Greece, to our modern-day self-initiation. For the time has come for us now to *realize,* or make real, that we have direct contact with the Source within the temple of our body.

We require no intermediaries other than Mother Nature's raw, organic foods as life energy of the Highest Order.

Everything in Mother Nature resonates with the force of the Divine, or spirit. Each raw, organic plant food carries and reflects spirit in its own way and conducts it to your central core. The more you are able to align with it and create your own resonance, the easier it will be to understand what Nature is doing and saying, and how She is evolving you to a higher octave within the light.

**All ancient wisdom traditions contain this key thought -
you are what you eat and have become what you think.**

The damage done however, can be undone. And this is the purpose of high vibrational foods. For they are our modern high vibrational medicine. The true nature and purpose of using high frequency food and elevating our thought frequencies is to purify our bodies and strengthen our much deteriorated nervous systems for the infusion of our spirit.

Stepping Out Of The Not-Self and Into The True-Self

It has been said that new wine cannot be poured into old bottles. Old bottles must first be washed clean and made ready as new. So, too, spirit cannot be poured into old, worn out, low vibrational bodies. It only awaits your commitment to your greater Self to uplift your body and consciousness to the higher vibrations of Light. You can turn inward to the Divine, or God-essence, within. This Force is always with you.

Raw, live salads and especially sprouts *ascension-initiate* your meal of high vibrational life force into your cells. Blessing opens the palm chakras, activating and opening the twelve body meridians, part of the ancient science of mudra. Your body then becomes the sacred connector point and accumulator of Heaven and Earth energies. Your table and tablecloth function as your altar and altar cloth for filling yourself with the fullness of Holy Presence. Our gratitude is spoken in our words of thanks and we align with the flow of One-ness.

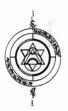

It is a little known fact here in the West what has long been known in the East, that certain foods and certain symbols provide openings for spiritual emergence. Zon-O-Ray and I have discovered how to shift the body's frequencies by the use of the high frequency food and the cosmic codes you find throughout this book. Both these modalities provide you with electromagnetic field nutrition which ensures that you can feel, and know, that this Force is *really* with you.

Hippocrates, the father of western medicine once said, "*Let food be your medicine and your medicine be your food.*" Our Prime Directive today is that high vibrational food becomes our high vibrational medicine. Our high vibrational medicine foods then open us into the high vibrational flow of One-ness. Via self-purification and self-initiation you demonstrate mastery of your *material nature* and your own transmutational release into the True Self you are, from the not-Self you once were. Your body is the laboratory for this experiment in Self-realization by Self- actualization.

The Virgin Birth of Self

A similar experiment was carried out by the Essenes. Sequestered on the banks of the Dead Sea for some two hundred years or more, they ate mostly raw foods and attuned themselves by meditation and prayer to prepare their bodies vibrationally so that one day, the high vibrational being known to us as Jesus, might take human birth through one of them. In Essence, we are modern-day Essenes and ours is the virgin birth of Self.

III. Ensuring The Force Is With You Through Alchemical Renewal

The Integration period (from 8 pm to 4 am) and the Elimination period (from 4am to noon) require a great deal of work and energy from the body. Digestion, from 12 noon to 8 PM, may require up to 60% of the body's energy reserves and even more if food is badly combined. Badly combined foods and toxic or dead foods leave you much like a dead battery, drained of life force. This makes it even harder to rejuvenate and regenerate. It takes an astonishing amount of energy to rebuild and repair existing deterioration in your body. Various researchers suggest that the body needs between five to ten times the nutritional support to build and repair than it does to maintain itself. Others suggest that nothing in the human body heals in less than three months and some say you need to add one month to that for each year of ill health!

When live, organic foods carrying life force are eaten, you feel light. That's because you are becoming light, enabled to be fed by and to carry the repatterning frequencies of light.

The ways in which foods are combined are of paramount importance in catalyzing life energy within your body.

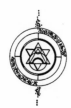

High Vibrational Foods are Your Perfect Energy Medicine

Food combining is actually based on a very simple, but little-known fact that starches or carbohydrates and proteins cannot be efficiently digested together in the stomach at the same time. Proteins require an acidic digestive secretion by the stomach while starches require an alkaline one. As you know from high school chemistry classes, when an acid and an alkali meet, they cancel each other out. In our stomach's case, digestion ceases.

Normally food should remain in the stomach for about three hours for the digestive process there. It then passes along into the small intestine. If the food is not suitably broken down in the gastric process, it will remain in the stomach for eight to ten hours, or more. Left this long, the undigested protein putrifies and the undigested starch ferments. The results are variously called gas, wind, acid indigestion, flatulence, heartburn, upset stomach, nausea, dizziness and on occasion, vomiting. Over time, chronic conditions result such as headaches, lethargy, skin eruptions, backaches, and so on.

In addition, when such spoiled food continuously moves through the digestive tract day after day, no nutrition is supplied to the body, whereas increasingly poisonous levels of toxemia are. Because we have unknowingly and unwittingly had this inculcated habit conditioned into our very psyches, it has become a *programme* affecting both our genes and our jeans. The medical term for this is autotoxemia, or self-poisoning. My term for it is the not–Self.

The vibrational result is that the lower and slower frequency domain of the intestines become open doorways for anaerobic parasites, bacterial and viral overgrowth and low level "entities" whose poisonous and addictive habits run you into the ground, both literally and figuratively. The first, second and third chakras become distorted and out of sync, and as sink holes, energetically attract lower entities and energies of like vibration. What we "put out," we "get back." We can very simply break the code, or signal marker, which has locked this part of our physical self into this self-destructive and dis-ease prone not-Self process. We need only start to eat meals with either one starch or one protein, but not both.

When these meals are preceeded by a large, raw organic salad too, existing toxemia is assisted to slowly exit the body. True to Hermetic traditions, this works from the top down to gently but effectively remove the "stuff" in the same sort of food-eating process that originally laid down the toxic sludge in the first place. As mentioned earlier, raw salads should comprise at least 50% of the weight, not the volume, of your lunch and dinner.

In this way, your food does, indeed, become your perfect medicine as Hippocrates stated ages ago. Nowadays we ring the update on this for our rapidly changing times by realizing that high vibrational food is our energy medicine and our energy medicine is our high vibrational food. We are led from within nowadays, too, in the initiate's process of self-purification within the temple of the body. We drop the not-Self through the right use of our free will to become our True Self. Organic foods "light" the initiate's path into self-mastery through evolutionary resonance. The following pages outline how you too, can give it a whirl.

Alchemical Formula #2
High Vibrational Foods Produce Alchemical Renewal by:

- observing the body's three daily cycles
- combining foods correctly
- the correct eating of fruit
- chewing correctly
- correct drinking
-

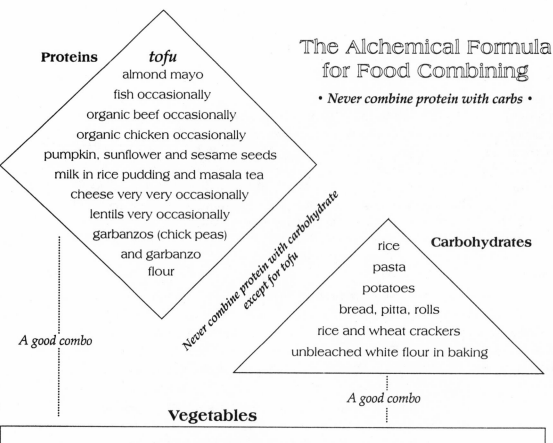

The Alchemical Formula for Food Combining

• *Never combine protein with carbs* •

Proteins

tofu

almond mayo

fish occasionally

organic beef occasionally

organic chicken occasionally

pumpkin, sunflower and sesame seeds

milk in rice pudding and masala tea

cheese very very occasionally

lentils very occasionally

garbanzos (chick peas)

and garbanzo
flour

Never combine protein with carbohydrate except for tofu

Carbohydrates

rice

pasta

potatoes

bread, pitta, rolls

rice and wheat crackers

unbleached white flour in baking

A good combo

A good combo

Vegetables

Avocados, cucumbers, bell peppers and tomatoes are botanically fruits.
Like all fruits when cooked, they acidify the body.

Non-Starch Vegetables

asparagus	kohlrabi
aubergine (eggplant)	leeks
broccoli	lettuce
brussels sprouts	okra (ladies fingers)
cabbage	onions
celery	parsley
chard	parsnips
chicory	radishes
cilantro (coriander)	spinach
courgettes (zucchini)	sprouts
collard greens	sprouted seeds
dandelion	summer squash
endive	crookneck squash
escarole	turnip
green beans	watercress
kale	zucchini

Vegetables with a slight Starch Content

artichokes	celery root
beets	corn
carrots	mushrooms
cauliflower	peas

The Alchemical Formula for Food Combining Is:
◦ **Protein should never be combined with carbohydrate** ◦

On the opposite page you will see three shapes. Proteins are listed in the diamond shape ◇, carbohydrates are listed in the triangular shape △ and veggies are listed in the square shape □.

With regard to food combining practices, the chart shows you that:

- any protein ◇ can always be combined with any and all veggies □
- any carb △ can also be combined with any and all veggies □
- any veggie □ can be combined with any other veggie □
- if you like sweet things for dessert, remember to include them in your protein and/or carbohydrate calculations

•

There are only two no-no's :

- Protein ◇ must never be combined with a carb △ with the one exception of tofu which is a vegetable protein and can combine with a carbohydrate.

- It is best to have just one protein at any given meal or just one carbohydrate at any given meal so that less energy is required by the digestive process and more energy can be given over to the necessary rebuilding and rejuvenating processes instead.

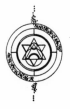

Avoiding Acidity and Overweight

In our western society most people are prone to acidic conditions. This is because toxicity is acidic. Acidic toxic waste in our body contributes to overweight. It has been said that the average American carries anywhere between 5 to 15 pounds (or more) of toxic intestinal sludge. If more toxicity goes into your system than can be eliminated each day, your thighs, buttocks, tummy, midsection, upper arms and double chin along with balding, cellulite, nervousness and dark circles under the eyes will bear silent witness to your problems. Your body further protects its internal organs by storing the by-products of incomplete digestion and uneliminated waste in the fatty tissue and the muscles, in all those very places listed above, where we least like to "bulge." In addition, water bloating is the body's way of neutralizing increasing toxic and acidic conditions. This also adds more "weight."

Here's a quick and simple test for acidity.

Do you know those gnawing "hunger" pangs which then prompt you to eat? Well, it's not hunger, but an acid condition of the stomach which is making itself apparent. When we put food in to satisfy our constant cravings, on the mistaken assumption that we're hungry, we just give the stomach a digestion job, diverting it from cleansing and clearing itself. Acidity results from the fermentation of food and the stomach's inability to digest it. Over time the system breaks down and secondary symptoms appear such as, rheumatism, diminished vision, "sour" disposition, night grinding of the teeth and parasites. So, instead of eating, cleanse your stomach by drinking water until the "hunger" pangs disappear.

You can also use Natrum Phosphoricum 6X, a Schuessler biochemic remedy, to help you neutralize chronic acidity until your new transformational food lifestyle kicks in. Your irritable, sour-puss, not-Self soon disappears and your bright and shiny new, True Self steps forth.

Good food combining, along with alkaline veggies and alkaline morning fruit meals, start to eliminate stored toxicity and acidity. Eliminating other acid-forming elements such as animal flesh, dairy, eggs, salt, cereals, wheat flour, grains, coffee, tea, soda, tobacco and alcohol will help, too.

In addition, drinking freshly squeezed lemon juice in water frequently throughout the day will help to strip out mucous. Freshly squeezed grapefruit juice actually helps to dissolve fat from the body as well. All fresh, raw fruit and vegetables neutralize acidity when eaten correctly.

Beauty, health, longevity, energy, happiness, normal weight and spiritual realizations such as increased intuition and inner knowing, emerge from the real Self like a butterfly from the distorted caterpillar of your not-Self.

You've got nothing to lose and nowhere to go, but up!

We've been there and done that and we'd like you to have the t- shirt, too!

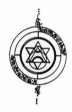

But, like we've said before, nothing is chiseled in stone.

Likewise for food combining. We basically followed the food combining principles, except when we didn't. We do however, follow our own inner knowing and our spirit no matter what. If we feel we are supposed to have a McDonalds hamburger, a coke, a coffee, a beer, a glass of champagne or whatever else, how we know what to do is this. We "check in" first and foremost, to get a "hit" We suggest you check this out for yourself to see how your spirit works with you.

Each being is unique. What we share with you in these pages is what worked for us. We share this data not as the one and only truth but as stimulation to your own inner knowing of what is yours to do for you.

Just as one man's meat is another's poison,
one man's ceiling is another man's floor.

•

Remember, too, that the cleaner and purer your body becomes, the better it can transmute toxic or "poisonous" foods. But you have to get it clean first!

•

Alchemical Formula #3
Food Combining Provides an Alchemical Formula for Self-Healing

Try the three formulae given in this chapter for just six weeks.
40 days is the magic number for initiating change. Lent is
40 days. Jesus spent 40 days in the desert. If you'd
like to see the results which you can achieve, and
the habits of a lifetime – or more – which you
can break, we suggest that you check
it out by religiously applying
the three formulae
given.

•

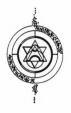

Einstein and subsequent physicists assure us that matter is born from energy and that energy is light. Energy, or light, has a dual nature. It can function as matter and it can function as light. This means that matter is frozen light. Our bodies are frozen light. Right now our bodies are simply thawing, into a higher energy expression of light.

All the ancient and modern alchemical formulae simply involve purifying our bodies and our thoughts for the body-mind-spirit eMergence into en-light-enment.

Of course, you already knew that and
this is merely a reminder.

o

If art is frozen music
And man is frozen light,
Our molecules are, of course, excited
To be eMailed right out of the night!

•

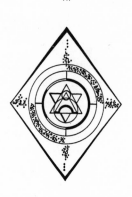

The Light Touch :

o

Some "Hands-On" Techniques for Restructured Field Effects

o

The Kiss of Light

o

The Kiss of Life

o

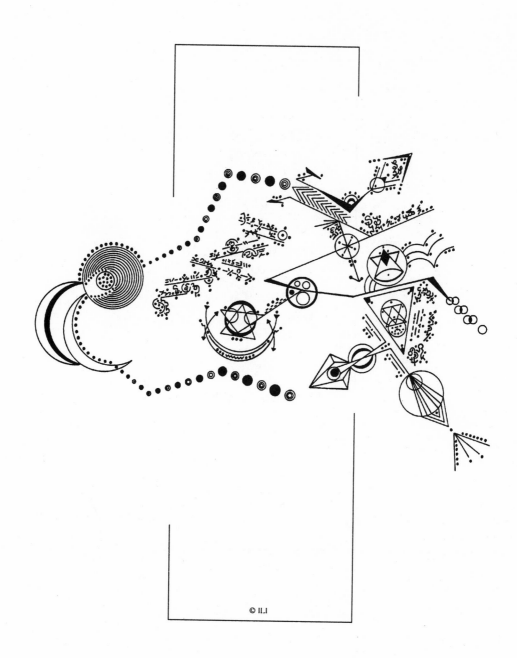

The Kiss of Light

Some Hands-On Techniques for Restructured Earth Field Effects

I. Food Preparation : Pulling in the Light

There are many ways to touch the divine, the divine within each of us. The art of the sushi chef is an active Zen meditation. It is one tao, or "way" to achieve "union with God." I came to know more about that in preparing the food as part of my own active Zen meditation programme. I had to wait for a "hit" on what to do. I had to listen "up." I had to tune in and turn on to the synergies formed by every being participating in each meal in order to prepare that meal for those beings.

Everything is cut and grated by hand. My utensils are simple and extremely minimal : a Kershaw cook's knife and a 4 and 1/2 inch serrated knife, a Japanese ginger grater, one small, fine Japanese vegetable grater and one coarse, a stainless steel garlic press and several serving spoons. I already had a couple of heavy stainless steel pots and a carbon steel wok. Aluminum is toxic, leaves residues in the body and is a known contributor to Alzheimer's disease. The only electricity I work with is via a small Braun hand blender. I use no dishwasher and cook with gas. With these few utensils I have prepared meals for up to 40 people. Anything can happen when you consciously step into the "light."

This "light" or cosmic energy comes through you to then be emitted in your conscious "hands on" technique. Via mudra, this energy in turn touches and evokes from within, each being contacting that sensitive, conscious cosmic essence vibrating within your food. It also further charges the atomic and subatomic spin rates. All you have to do is to be aware, awake and aware of what you truly are capable of. This food programme was simply my learning curve and now I can pass it on to you. What I realize more and more nowadays is how the "ripple effect" creates new vibratory waves. Everyone is becoming more and more sensitive to energy streams. Like a stone in a pond, the ripple effect energetically affects everyone who comes into contact with it.

In one workshop in Munich, participants were each holding a vegetable, tuning in to what they might hear, or feel or see. One woman was so overwhelmed that her broccoli had actually telepathically responded, that in her joy and surprise she forgot what it had said. This sort of experience alters our lives and brings a depth of new meaning to our emerging new reality in which everything, every single thing, is alive, intelligent and part of the Divine One-ness.

II. Eating : Ingesting the Light

Eating this high vibrational food became an active meditation too. Everyone on the programme looked forward to it, took time for it, and put everything else aside to focus on communing with it. A One-ness, one could say. This occurred completely spontaneously. Many felt strongly that the food "spoke" to their bodies. Of course it actually does. Mother Nature communes with us constantly. Everyone attunes to "Mother's" Force, each in their own unique way. This is what is meant by Holy Communion with the Divine.

Chewing is also a meditation. Knowing that you are light and infusing your body with more light is what it's all about. When you chew, or do, with that "in mind", you are engaging with what is known as a **restructured field effect**. This is a new technology of consciousness we are all becoming aware of. It's the focused consciousness of the universal mind field, focused at one single point – **You**. And that focus of your mind in resonance with "Divine Mind" exponentially raises your vibrations, setting a benchmark for others to follow the energetic pathway you are cutting towards the light.

You change or restructure your field when you change or restructure your conscious thoughts and actions. Your "restructured field effects" affect all those who touch it. It's as simple as that. As Mahatma Ghandi once said:
"I must first BE the change I want to see in this world."

III. Blessing : Anchoring the Light

Blessing the food naturally arose as I went along. I just began to feel the life force and its flow. Then at some point I found myself just naturally talking to the intelligence within the various vegetal life forms. The teams, as I call my awareness of my other dimensionality, once showed me how to vitalize a nearly dead supermarket cauliflower. When I held it in both hands and tuned in, I found myself bursting out loud *"Oh, you poor thing!"* I recall a Kirlian photo I once saw of an ordinary glass of tap water, unblessed and then blessed by a laying on of hands. The energy field of the blessed water danced and scintillated. It looked like joy to me. In blessing this cauliflower I "sensed" its response as upliftment.

What telepathically formed in my mind went something like this : *"I call upon the Overlighting force of this cauliflower and ask that it be filled with life force as appropriate for the highest good of all concerned."* I then thanked it for its purposefulness in participating with me and all the others on the programme in the co-creation of Heaven on Earth. And then I felt I should let it know the form that its participation was going to take, as a cauliflower curry. After that I found I telepathically communicated with all other foods to thank them for the part they would be playing in each meal and asked them to prepare to be cut. I also let them all know that I had finally found the finest and best Japanese knives for this purpose, my *Kershaws*.

Prior to becoming part of the InterGalactic Café, I used to give a little inner prayer of thanks to my food for its purposeful assistance with me in the co-creation of Heaven on Earth before eating it. So I guess that gave a natural impetus to my ever growing awareness during the preparing of it. Blessing is a praise. In this case, for a job well done by them!

IV. Mudra: Filling Yourself, Your Food and Others With Light

Someone once said that the science of ritual or sacred ceremony recreates universal order out of our individual chaos. In Buddhist and other Eastern cultures, Mudra, or ceremonial hand gestures, have a wide variety of meanings and applications. This is why they are included in dance, statues of deities and in yogic postures. Everyone energetically benefits from them, even if not consciously so.

All twelve bodily acupuncture meridians end in the finger tips. While modern instruments can now register just some of the many subtle energies entering and emanating from the hands, and especially the fingers, all ancient cultures have known about them and taught their uses and applications for eons.

We use the hands in our food preparation. The more that we can use our hands consciously and in full awareness of our powers, the more we can infuse our food and our drink with life force energies to get well. No kitchen machine can ever replace or replicate this. In fact, the electromagnetic field of our 60 cycle machines along with our microwave ovens destroy the very subtle energies of evolutionary resonance we now require.

Our food and drink are merely the carriers of life force energies. Without the pranic forces of Mother Nature which they carry, we would die. Life force is light. Light is a high vibrational energy. It is the "ether" or "etheric Light" which interpenetrates all of space. Physicists tell us that we are, actually, 98% space and only 2% matter. So we are filled with this etheric life force energy, or chi, in 98% of our bodily being. Our twelve meridians form our etheric interface and the flow conductors of this life force energy, or chi, into and out of our bodies. You can open your palm chakras to radiate and flow the highest of subtle energies received from the crown chakra and those above, down through your body and out of your hands and finger tips.

How do you do this? You just intend to do so and watch the results, both in your food and in yourself. When you know that you are spirit having a human experience, there is nothing you cannot do. Your words are a Mantra or sacred sound. Your gestures are Mudra or sacred gestures of light emanation. Such is the sacred law, that you and what you do are sacred because you decide that it is, you say that it is and you act that it is. And so it is! Easy isn't it? Thought, word and deed are sanctified and purified and the energy from the sacred domains or higher energy dimensions flow down through our thoughts, words and deeds and out onto this third energy domain, or dimension. *As above, so below.*

So, bless your food and pray, opening your palm chakras and the finger acupuncture points to place energies that can heal and transform within your foods or "food vehicles" which you prepare in your kitchen. This is the true meaning of sacred communion. It brings a wholly, holy new meaning to your kitchen as an alchemical altar, your food as a sacred offering and your ingestion of its light as a divine sacrament. For this is the body and blood of the Divine becoming manifest in your body and blood. You are a divine extension and manifestation of the Divine Mudra, empowered to go with this flow. Michaelangelo captured this in The Creation of Adam on the ceiling of the Sistine

Chapel. Take a moment now, if you'd care to, and just conjure up in your mind's eye God's hand gesture or mudra as He infuses Adam with life. Made in the "image and similitude" of the Divine Source, we are empowered to create in Divine Love too, as stewards of this planet and all its life forms. We are all learning now to come into our Divine God-given inner power.

V. Mudra of Light: The Hands of Prayer

When Universal Life Force energy or chi, moves through us without obstruction, we are in perfect union or at–One–ment with One–ness. However, the stresses and strains of daily living often predispose us to physical, mental, emotional, and electro-magnetic field disturbances of one sort or another. All too often we are not even aware of the resulting obstructions and blockages in our auric field or body until we start feeling "all bent out of shape." This is the moment to stop everything we are doing and "lighten" the load of human self by reconnecting to our Divine Self.

One of the most powerful mudras, the Hands of Prayer, is also known worldwide. In a way it's really a total body/mind/spirit harmonizer since it re-establishes balance and that sense of deep inner peace and One-ness with the universe. This is the time-honored self-help mudra of the hands in prayer.

All ancient cultures recognized and used this ritual gesture or mudra, not as our Western religions do as a symbolic, supplicant's gesture to an external and wrathful "god," but as a practical, yet simple, "hands on" way to reconnect with the flow and harmony of the Universe and that self-healing which results. Of course, as in all things, it is the actual intention you fill it with that switches on the light and makes it work. Empty rituals are just that, empty.

You can choose to hold this mudra as the hands in prayer. You can also alternately press the thumb of one hand into the centre of the palm or palm chakra of the other hand. You can do whichever version you choose until the chaos in your universe is reconnected and harmonized with the flow and Love of the heart of Universal order. It is the intent which helps carry you there, the carrier wave, so to speak. The peaceful feeling is the indicator light of the vibrational shift back into your true home, the Higher Light, popping back into your true self as it were.

Modern day stresses cause brain imbalance. One hemisphere becomes dominant, usually the left analytical part of the brain. The right hemisphere of the brain connects us to spirit, or our True Self. Eastern and Middle-Eastern cultures which still read from right to left, for example, retain a truer connection to spirit because of that. Our brain can be considered to be "whole," and functional as an instrument of spirit, only when the impulses from our highest Self are received by the right hemisphere and processed by the left brain in harmony with the right brain.

The computer is a good metaphor and outpicturing for this. The left side of the brain is like the hardware. The right is like the zip drive. Spirit, the causal body or highest aspect of Self, is the operator. An individual's life expression on this plane of experience is the print-out. If the hardware of the left brain tries to be the operator, there can be numerous glitches in the program. Hal, the computer in the movie "2001," provides the perfect example of this. When we find ourselves in overload or under stress on this plane of experience, the left brain usually tries to take over, like Hal the computer. Life on planet Earth subsequently runs amok on this program. So when we say "get with the programme," now we can know what we truly mean. We mean, "get with the higher programme."

To "get with the programme" faster, you can place your hands together in the Universal Mudra of Light. Then describe in the air an infinity sign, or a figure 8 lying sideways. Do this from right to left, in slow, lazy but wide gestures, until you feel a sort of "click." It's a feeling that you've got yourself together again and things have "clicked" into place. Usually 8 to 10 or 12 times is sufficient to rebalance your brain to whole brain functioning and in line with Universal or Divine Order. Then its universal light flows through you, without impedance, once more.

In this way you are learning to bend light in service both to your Highest Self and to this world. You become the stone dropped into this world's pond. You are making new waves. The ripple effect is a quickening for the times ahead.

To remind myself of my own connectedness to the Divine, I also have a small shrine in my kitchen. Quan Yin and the Buddha sit on their respective little altar flames with their hands in mudra gestures of *protection* and *touching* the earth, respectively.

These altars, shrines, deities and rituals serve to remind us again and again of who we really are and our own inner power. They remind us to release that power first, to master and benefit ourselves. Then we are truly able to be of benefit to this world through bending our light and the universal light to world Service, just as our forefathers Buddha and Jesus did in service to the great Divine Mother of us all.Crystals, candles and flowers, among other things, enhance this precious, little space.

VI. Blessed by the Light : Welcomed into the Light

The mind does not feel or experience. The body and emotions do. As I see it, the trick is to not be tricked by the mind's thinking kind of knowing. The trick is to experience knowing in the body and in the emotions, or a feeling kind of knowing. Knowing is a feeling. When the body and emotions are open along with the mind, all goes forward according to plan – The plan. In this I feel the food blesses us, encourages us and most definitely lifts us up. Everyone on the programme could feel the light.

This is of course, what is true for us. That this is so you can only experience for yourself. Thinking does not make it so. *Experiencing* it makes it real and unmistakable and true for *you.* The truth is, it is only what you experience and what is true for you that matters. The evidence is that your True Self within emerges.

Oxygen is an Intelligence

Oxygen is an intelligence. It is in service to life. It is in service to the human body's transfigurational processes now squarely underway. Oxygen serves life both graphically and holographically. Lakes in Eastern Europe, dead for decades, are being revivified by it. The bio-energetics or the patterns of the frequencies of oxygen ALONE are enough. These frequency patterns of oxygen, but not oxygen itself, are simply introduced into the dead waters. These metal plates carrying the frequency patterns of oxygen work like a yantra does. A yantra is simply a sacred frequency pictorialized.

Regeneration and new life return to the waters in a matter of months.

Another such healing pattern or yantra is Zon-O-Ray's **TransFiguration Chakra Balancer**. It's a template of high frequency healing vibrations pictorialized for use in this dimension. It functions with each individual uniquely. It works to support your human body's evolution into the next level of expression as light body. For more information, please see pages 148 and 149 in the section entitled "Glimpses Into the Invisible" at the end of the book.

Eating : The Kiss of Life

Raw foods contain oxygen. Processed, chemicalized, dead foods do not. Naturally death does not give life. Life gives life. Electron rich oxygenated food and water in your body unlocks and releases the evolutionary potentials pre-designed into that human body. You are not that body. You are the consciousness in that body which is here to assist its transition into light body.

Oxygenation provides the major fuel for self-purification, self-healing and ultimately for light body lift-off.

Breathing : The Kiss of Life

You can oxygenate your body more by breathing more deeply, using the diaphragm muscle. Most people breathe shallowly from the upper chest, a symptom of fright. This fear is fed into the cells and as a consequence the auric field collapses. High vibrational information has a tough time getting through that. Breathing deeply and oxygenated food and water relax the body. The auric or bio-electromagnetic field expands again. The life force frequencies can then pass through the acupuncture meridian interface to feed the etheric or electromagnetic field and subsequently the cells of the body. Fear is exhaled in the sigh of relief. Exercising oxygenates the body opening our auric field to the "nourishment" of subtle energies which we all require in our spirit-matter evolvement. We find the Tibetan exercise rites in the book, *Ancient Secrets of the Fountain of Youth* by Peter Kelder, to be helpful for breathing , exercising, and correcting chakra spin.

Exercise : Dancing with the Kiss of Life

Meditation has now been widely researched in the West and recognized as an aerobic "exercise," or oxygen builder. Conditions which thrive on a lack of oxygen are anaerobic and are thus dis-ease producing. In the presence of oxygen, however, anaerobic dis-ease conditions dissipate and eventually disappear. Exercise, oxygenating food and drink, proper food combining, blessing, mudra and meditation - all aerobically improve the oxygen levels in the body. The chi, or life essence which all these modalities carry, illumines or "lights" the body. This is the process of physical en-light-enment. It's a faster vibration from the "frozen light" of our body matter which is fast becoming an incandescent body of light.

Many people have occasionally experienced a chi rush through sports activity or peak "high" moments in their life experience. Recently we found a Japanese machine which delivers a chi rush or a chi "high" when doing what is called the lying down exercise.

Almost everyone knows, or has heard it said that a brisk walk of 30 to 45 minutes every day is enough exercise to maintain health and oxygenation and therefore longevity. This chi machine delivers the effect of walking 10,000 steps in just 15 minutes and while lying down, as mentioned before. This is a marvelous way to exercise during prolonged periods of bad weather or late at night after a long day at the office. Details on the chi machine which we found to be most helpful for combining meditation, oxygenation and exercise can be found on page 150 at the back of the book.

Drinking : The Kiss of Life

Water is H_2O. Hydrogen peroxide contains extra oxygen - H_2O_2. We tested oxygenated water by diluting hydrogen peroxide in purified drinking water. We now use about 7 drops of 35% food grade hydrogen peroxide in each gallon of drinking water. Pint sized bottles are available from our local health food shop.

If you cannot locate any 35% food grade hydrogen peroxide in your area, 3% from the drug store will do fine. Please do check the label carefully to ensure there are no stabilizers or any other ingredients listed which would make the hydrogen peroxide unsuitable for internal use.

The skin is a large absorptive organ. We spritzed our bodies at first with a half 3% and half water mixture, rubbing it onto our damp bodies after showering. We also used this 1-1/2% solution as a mouth wash and gargle.

Part of our mutational process involved detoxing via the mouth. For this we also found the Schuessler biochemic tissue salt Ferrum Phosphoricum 6X very useful. These soft tablets melted into sore and disturbed areas of the mouth, oxygenating the cells by homeopathically boosting the iron in the blood. Homeopathics are truly energy medicines. They treat the etheric body first which, in turn, benefits the physical body. There is no actual substance in a homeopathic remedy, only Mother Nature's vibration or "energetic signature" of the original substance.

The Kiss of Life for Foods

Detoxing and Oxygenating Foods

We experimented with soaking chemically grown fruit and vegetables in oxygenated water. The information in Elizabeth Brown's book *The UnMedical Miracle – Oxygen** provided a starting point. Then I just "checked in" to ask what was appropriate on each occasion after that.

> In these as in all other situations, we suggest you "check in" with
> your spirit for what's right for you. Each being is unique.
> What serves us may not serve you.

Oxygenating Salads

Commercially grown lettuce was first washed and then spritzed with oxygenated water to carry more oxygen into the salads. Unused washed leaves and salad leftovers kept far longer in the fridge without wilting after they'd been spritzed first in this way.

Oxygenating Sprouts

Eventually I found that the sprouts could be spritzed during growth rather than being rinsed in ordinary tap water. They grew very quickly without any mustiness. In the fridge sprouts have kept for an incredible two weeks or more in a zip lock bag when periodically spritzed too.

- A salad spinner covered with a double layer of cheesecloth and kept in a cupboard is perfect for sprouting. You can also use Mason jars or any clean large glass jars you may already have.

- Sunflower sprouts with their two juicy green little leaves keep extremely well in the fridge in an airtight tupperware lined with paper kitchen towel.

Superoxygenation : A Great Big Kiss of New Life

If oxygen is a vital life enhancer, superoxygenation is more so. Spirit burns more brightly in the body as debris is removed. All of the beings on the InterGalactic Café programme experienced break throughs in all sorts of ways. Both the food and oxygenation feed your light beingness, the real you in the body.

> This is the evidence of the "Mother" Force of Nature at work –
> the kiss of new life.

o

*Inidianola, WA: Drelwood Comns., 1991.

Oxygen is the Greatest Detoxifier on the Planet and the Fuel for Light Body Lift-Off

"The best tool I had in playing Spock was...to look for the differences...and celebrate them.

I had decided that the Vulcans were a peculiar race, with peculiar powers and that much of that emanated from their hands.

The Vulcans have an energy that comes off their fingertips...

I was able to call upon this... in coming up with the four finger split down–the–middle greeting. It is in reality a Jewish rabbinical blessing, but it seemed quite appropriate."

Leonard Nimoy –
Star Trek Memories by William Shatner with Chris Kreski
New York: HarperCollins, 1993, p. 131.

"We found out that when you drink hydrogen peroxide in your water, it goes into your stomach and in 13 seconds it will be out at the ends of your fingers."

Father Willhelm in
O₂xygen Therapies by Ed McCabe
Morrisville, NY: Energy Publications, 1989

"How much do we breathe daily?

The average person consumes 6 to 8 pounds of oxygen, 4 pounds of food and 2 pounds of water. More oxygen goes into our bodies than the other two combined. I would say oxygen is important."

Ed McCabe –
O₂xygen Therapies
Morrisville, NY: Energy Publications, 1989

"The very thought patterns that are associated with negativity and depression produce toxins in the body that increase the need for detoxifying oxygen . . . Hydrogen peroxide is 94% oxygen. . . Oxygen is the greatest detoxifier known to man."

Dr. Kurt Donsbach –
Oxygen, Oxygen, Oxygen
Tulsa, OK: Rockland Corporation, 1994

And talking about lift-off, rocket fuel is 90% hydrogen peroxide!

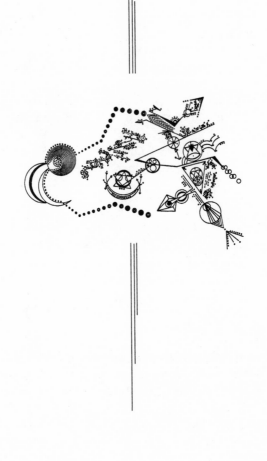

The InterGalactic Clinic :

Therapeutics

I
Some Cleansing and Clearing Technologies

II
There IS Light At The End of The Tunnel

III
Look Homeward, Angel

IV
Let There Be Light, And There IS Light

•

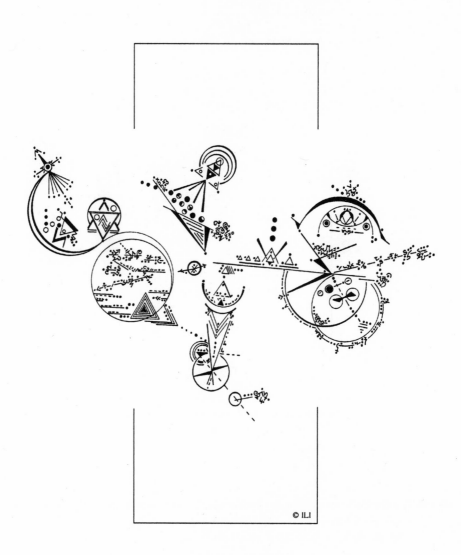

I. Some Cleansing and Clearing Technologies

Introduction

Although we can be purified by fire, baptism by water is a lot easier. Certain cleansing and clearing techniques assist light body integration. Here are a few tips which may help.

Do you know what free radicals are ?

"I keep reading that free radicals are a part of aging, as though this is normal! It's not normal. Just because we see it happen doesn't mean it's normal. It may be average, do you follow? Average meaning it happens. But it doesn't mean it's a normal happening.

It's a simple thing really because stress creates it. And, if you're in a contaminated environment, you don't get enough oxygen with its negative ion. Wherever you can get oxygen, you get negative ions. These can replenish the negative ions so your positive ion, which is the free radical, will not do its damage.

Cold showers help also. Showers are far better than baths. The refreshment you get from a shower is the refreshment not so much from the tingle on your skin or the circulation of your blood, but it's from the radiation of negative ions."

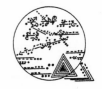

Dr. Valerie V. Hunt –
The Human Energy Field and Health

- Tepid showers are best. A hot shower followed by a cold rinse for as long as you can bear it will energize. Oxygenate further with 1-1/2% up to 3% hydrogen peroxide rubbed well into the skin after showering.

Chlorine and fluoride in tap water actually depletes the body's oxygen.

Hydrogen peroxide on the other hand,
superoxygenates the cells through the skin.

"Chlorine destroys vitamins and other beneficial factors in the body as it is absorbed through the skin into the bloodstream. Hot tubs and pools become health rejuvenators and disease fighters when treated with hydrogen peroxide instead of chlorine which is a real downer."

Elizabeth Baker –
The UnMedical Miracle – Oxygen
Indianola, WA: Drelwood Comns., 1991.

• **Environmental Tip :** An uncovered glass or small bowl of water kept by your head at night will absorb psychic debris and toxic fallout from your body and auric field while you sleep.

Hydrogen Peroxide "Works"

Hydrogen peroxide is manufactured via plant photosynthesis. So raw organic chlorophyll - containing food has lots of oxygen.

Hydrogen peroxide "works" by removing electrons from microorganisms. In the process the micro-organism is effectively killed while water (H_2O) and more importantly oxygen (O_2) is freed for light body fuel.

The frequencies or energy fields of oxygen carry their high cosmic vibrations into the recesses of each cell and its DNA, infusing the light body with light and acting as the fuel for that light body's release.

Spiritual Hygiene : The Violet Flame Cleanser

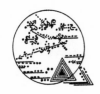

Whnever you are dropping density of any kind, this technique helps. Do it several times a day if necessary. Visualize the violet flame of transmutation and the silver ray of Grace mixing together to form a beautiful iridescent violet. Then see it pouring into your physical body and filling it. Then bring it through the emotional, mental, and spiritual bodies separately. Also, place sea salt into your bath water and invoke the rays. Wash your clothes and bedlinens with a handful of sea salt, to remove energetic residue. Because you do most of your clearing in your sleep, call in these rays to transmute the old energies as you make your bed.You'll feel so much better.

Tashira Tachi-ren –
What is Lighbody?
(Lithia Springs, GA: New Leaf, 1999), p 87.

Lavender Soap

We found Dr. Bronner's Lavender Soap to be an aromatic and soothing help to us. A beautiful old legend has it that lavender's particular mission is as a messenger to assist humanity in its return to our starry galactic home.

• **Environmental Tip :** Sea salt and a few drops of pure Lavender essential oil in your bath help to cleanse and clear the auric field of toxic thought patterns.

The Human Energy Field : A New Model of Being Human

"My research in this area has been done over the last 22 years. Before that I was a square physiology researcher. Then, all of a sudden, I saw the light. And I saw things happening to human beings that could not be explained in the old physiology. So what did I do? I went to southeast Asia and I studied. I went to China. I went to Japan. I looked. I watched. And I came back and changed my entire research.

I'm going to show you a videotape done with regular cameras and enhanced with computer enhancement. It is the human auric field depicted for those who are not normally able to see a human auric field.

We had this man stay with this variety of junk food for about 20 minutes. In that 20 minutes his whole field was affected by the junk food in exactly the same way had he eaten and digested it.

The same thing is true with health foods which are here seeds and grains. He stayed there and meditated with his hands over it. Notice the difference in the glow that came to his body as a result of the transaction with living things.

I did this primarily for educational purposes so that people could see things which they have no idea even exist."

"... You can get a dynamic energy field by your own thought processes. The energy field is much more dynamic in the heart. It's much more dynamic than the brain is..."

"... You don't have to go through great and horrendous things. You have to have a life in which you constantly, **constantly feed your electro–magnetic field.** You don't have to keep shocking it. You don't have to have the constant medications that many of us are using. Instead, stabilize the field. This makes the responsibility yours. You have to assume your responsibility.

So, like brushing your teeth and taking a shower, we must also learn how to nourish this part of ourselves."

Dr. Valerie V. Hunt –
The Human Energy Field and Health

Clearing the energy field of the crystallized karmic cobweb of vows from the human and off-planet genetic lineage

Many times, astral entities will intrude on our fields. Whether conscious or unconscious, we make agreements with them when we have moments of fear or need. These entities will attach themselves to us, usually promising some aspect of ourselves comfort in exchange for living vicariously through us. These exchanges are almost never worth it, as the astral entity is just as subject to distortion and the illusion of polarity as are beings of the 3rd dimension. They often feed on addictions of various types, be they substances or people. Some really enjoy anger and violence, and will spur arguments and feed off karmic situations, adding to the intensity of the karma. Sometimes, relationships between people are actually relationships between the entities attached to them! It is always a benefit to release these beings into the Light, so they can move on to their next stage of development and you can be free of their influence. The Entity Release is a good practice in any "Spiritual Hygiene" program. Some people do the Release on a regular basis, just to be sure no entities have "sneaked" into their fields. *Please be aware, you can only realease any agreements that you yourself have with these entities. You cannot release agreements for other people...*

Call for assistance: "Archangel Michael please bring down the tunnel of Light. Ariel, Azrael and Aru-Firi, please assist. I break any and all agreements or contracts, both conscious and unconscious, that I have made, anyone in my body has made, or anyone in my genetic lineage has made, with any astral entities, thoughtforms, demons, dark forces, elementals, aliens or boogies. Please go into the tunnel, we will take you home."

From the moment you begin an entity release, assume that feelings or thoughts may not be your own. Boredom, spaciness, resistance, "this stuff never works," anger, aches and pains, and grief may all be coming from the entities. Identify them and send them on i.e. "entity holding resistance, go into the Light!" Toning is very helpful to ease their release. When you feel clear or lighter, ask Michael to take the tunnel back to the Fifth Dimension.

Tashira Tachi–ren –
What is Lightbody?
(Litihia Springs, GA: New Leaf, 1999), pp. 88-89.

- We've used this technique, lots. It "works" like a circuit breaker. The human genetic code is opened, allowing you access to that 99% of so far unused DNA codicils, now coming on line for the divine new you!

Don't Drink Fluoridated Water

"The level of adenotriphosphates is lowered because of fluoride. When the body burns food, it stores the energy in a substance called ATP, or adenotriphosphates. . . . What does that mean ? If you've been drinking fluoridated water for a period of time, you are going to have less oxidative reactions (a lessened ability to burn food to produce energy). Therefore more diseases of all kinds – and less energy to fight them with.

Don't drink fluoridated water !"

Dr. Kurt Donsbach –
O₂xygen Therapies by Ed McCabe
Morrisville, NY: Energy Publications, 1989

Science Fiction is Actually Science Fact–ion

Perhaps *"Star Trek's"* phenomenal quarter century success is simply due to its sci-fi reminder of our own mandate and sci–fact mission in being here.

For we too, are in fact, here to explore new worlds and go where no human has ever gone before.

No wonder we wept when ET phoned home!
It hasn't always been easy!

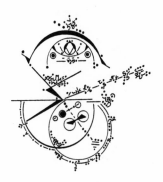

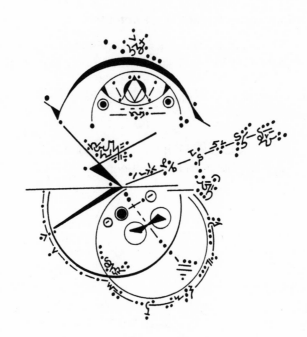

II. There IS Light at the End of the Tunnel !

Is There Really A Heaven ?

A lot of people ask, *"If there really is a Heaven, what's it like?"* Well there are plenty of modern day messengers whose mission is to provide us with this very data. These near death experiences (or NDE's) are more aptly called by those experiencing them, "real life experiences." This certainly reflects that life here on Earth is indeed more illusion than real when you know the difference !

Many books about NDE's have been written. Yet it is the childrens' experiences which are the most moving. When you read them, you cannot help but feel moved by their eloquent simplicity. **Except you become as little children, you cannot enter the kingdom of Heaven.**

All such experiences by adults and children alike, have the one, same thing in common. They all describe going down a tunnel and emerging in the light. In this light they float. It's filled with love and friends and family and joy and peace. It's not the rational mind type of understanding or knowing. It's the **feeling knowing** of being peace. It's the "peace that passeth all understanding."

All the data collected and now present in the human body or our cell suit let's call it, knows only death. These little crystals or crystallizations are full of the resonant experiences of being here on Earth. So the various experiences of NDE'ers are termed by those not experiencing them as "near death" experiences. In addition, these sort of doom and gloom perspectives naturally arise out of this cellularly recorded sense of loss collectively experienced and recorded at **this** end of the tunnel. The myriad memories of separation that have been the collective archetypical experience of **bodily life** over millenia here on Earth in cell suits, arises from this sense of separation and loss.

Now, we enter, we who are not these bodies, but the spiritual essence in these bodies. We have come into these bodies to take them home, into the light and that real life that so many NDE'ers are now busily and actively reporting on. This is something that these cellular bodies have never experienced before. Each being is unique. So each being will do this uniquely. *"What on Earth is happening"* these bodies may say. And you'll go, *"No, not on Earth. We're going to Heaven. Heaven on this Earth."* You see, we're going to explore new worlds where no human bodies have ever gone before. We're going home, into the Light.

But the real task we're also fulfilling is this. All the genetic ancestors and predecessors contributing to each unique human body's "cell suit" make up gets to go along for the ride. This is why the body is so important. All the source genetics are in all the earth bodies' DNA. And America is the gene pool of this world as well as of many other worlds. Salvation IS physical, truly.

We Hold These Truths To Be Self Evident

Earth is a kind of central plug. When we pull this plug on Earth, all the ancestral, genetic contributors both on and off planet go down the tunnel and into the light with us, as part of the ride. It's even better than Disney World. What's more, your ticket to ride is free. It's been imprinted in your DNA so no matter what you did, you couldn't lose it.

The founding fathers of these United States, this Federation of human genes, have some pretty moving things to say about this mission. "In God We Trust" they say. How to touch and energetically imprint this on people? Well, why not imprint this faith and trust on every bit of currency current. A current runs through you, right?

The US one dollar bill has a huge ONE. What does this ONE stand for? *Novus Ordo Seclorum* or, new world order. There's a pyramid on the one dollar bill which appears nowhere else. The apex is ascending in luminous light and contains one large all-seeing eye. This let's us know we are not alone and in deed, some One does watch over us.

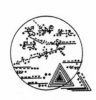

We hold these truths to be self evident, that all beings are created equal whether rocks, dolphins, dinosaurs, birds, bees, flowers, trees, men, women or androgyns, and have the right to life, liberty and the pursuit of happiness both for themselves and on behalf of all those other galactic orders here present which they may uniquely and individually represent on this journey back to the source.

Tunnel Vision

If you'd like to send a few care packages on into the light, there is a technique or technology which brings new 5th dimensional meaning to the 3rd dimensional expression of tunnel vision. It "works" like this.

Let's say you take the vow breaking seriously and you start removing limiter or inhibitor devices which are hampering your next moves into light body. So you identify, say, that your body is afraid to ascend and your mind and emotions have some serious considerations around what your mom or your partner or your neighbors might think as you "go through the roof." OK. So you break the vows around that as outlined earlier.

Then you close your eyes and visualize or feel the tunnel like the NDE'ers describe. At the far end is this incredibly bright light. Pour into that light in your own unique way, whatever debris you notice is in the tunnel after being shattered by your vow break. You can make tonal sounds, fast forward the speed if there's a lot of stuff hanging around and hanging out. See, or feel, all of it completely dissolve into the light.

Set Your Seal

Set your seal on all that debris by toning in a tonal language or sound intonations which "feel" right for you to express. It doesn't have to be loud or wake the neighbors. Subtlety remember, is powerful. And you are learning how to command the subtlety of the universal mind field. In the 5th dimension things happen because you say so. We're in a training programme which is focusing on recycling the matter here on earth so it can be remattered, so to speak. It works on your say so.

Whenever you feel doubt, anger, fear, grief, etc etc etc, look within, find the vow motivating it and set it a–light. Kiss it goodbye. With a mere wave of your hand you can wave it all goodbye without even lifting your finger. It's as easy as falling off an intergalactic log.

But hear this. These little lost energies will thank you for it.
Trust, and take your leap into faith.
We're all dancin' out of the night and into the light.
So put on your dancing shoes
and get ready for some **serious** dancin' guys!

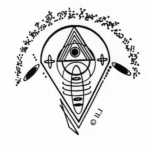

III. Look Homeward, Angel !

Each being is unique, so each will have a unique transmutational process. We offer what follows as broad brush strokes or guide lines of various possibilities. At the same time it has to be said that we have spent the last 4 years intensively gathering this data. Many of you reading this book may find in these rapidly accelerating times that for you this translates to only a matter of days, hours or even minutes. And, we are rapidly approaching a time in which whatever you participate with as real, will be real, and in your face in nanoseconds. So, you can look upon this time as a rapid fire introduction and learning curve between this now, and that 5th dimensional now which will soon be this now.

5D Training Mode

So, we are basically suggesting that you prepare yourselves to be fully in this training programme. Firstly, you assist all processes mightily if you alter your outlook from what many would term what's "wrong" with whatever is happening, to a single minded and determined focus on what's "right" about each and every thing that occurs. For example, diarrhea is a common occurence as cleansing and clearing out of cellular debris takes place.

Now you can look at it like this – it's an exciting clearing out of density and other old doo-doo / poo poo / ca ca or shit so higher vibrations can occupy the space being vacated for that purpose. Drink plenty of liquids, and bath/shower/swim/hot tub/jacuzzi or whatever, often. Water and oxygen assist in soothing and smoothing out all cleansing processes. Whining, moaning and complaining just don't cut it any more. Allowing, accepting and being open let the new **substantiation** into the cells. First the new vibrations have to seat themselves. Then they become operative. This is a cellular **trans-substantiation** process.

You are a walking, talking, real, live living miracle. To become a fully fledged miracle, you gotta dump a little doo-doo, yes?! Why not celebrate that. At the same time, know too, that nausea, discomforts or whatever else will pass as quickly as you let it! It passes quicker when you take your focus off the discomforts and plant your focus firmly on the light being you are becoming because of it.

Universal Law Numero Uno

Whatever you focus on you get more of. Want more shit !?!? You're certainly welcome to it! Want more Heaven? Fantastic! You're not alone there. Let's get more of it here. Let's live as if it's landing, right here, right now, right before our very eyes. We live that. **So can you!** Like the Native Americans say, walk your talk. Now IS the time. Talk is cheap. Actions speak louder than words.

Life IS NEVER Meant to be A Struggle

So, if yours is, you can break that vow, send it down the tunnel and into the light. Now, use your focus technique to focus on the universe providing everything you need. It knows you're here. After all, you asked it if you could come. You certainly know the technique works wonderfully. After all, when you focused on life being a struggle, it sure was, wasn't it?

OK, so now you know the principle works. And you know how it works. So you can now focus on life being full of ease and grace. See it. Feel it. Taste it. Touch it. Smell it. Everywhere.

Pegasus Products does a wonderful starlight elixir. We found it extremely useful. It works. It works vibrationally. It's called *Zeta Tauri* and it's for pattern breaking. When you focus your attention on breaking these vows and getting on with your vision of Heaven on Earth, that vision really starts manifesting. Check it out. Starlight elixirs are available from Pegasus Products, P. O. Box 228, Boulder, CO 80306, (800)527-6104 in the USA, (970)667-3019 ouside the USA, email: starvibe@indra.net, website: www.pegasusproducts.com.

Co-Creating with the Universe

By now you must be seeing that you are, in deed, a co-creator with the universe. You always were. You still are. You always will be. So . . . what's been co-created on Earth is done. It's over. Whew! Now that's done, what's next? You are co-creating your part of the new world. No one else can do this for you. You've got a vital piece of this new world coded in your genes. The time is here to let it out. It isn't like a bunch of us are going to co-create Heaven on Earth and you get a free condo. UH UH. No, no, no! I co-create my bit. You co-create your bit. He co-creates his bit. She co-creates her bit. It co-creates its bit. The whole is more than the sum of the myriad parts. All parts are key. You are the key. Get the picture!?

Grace

So this brings us to the subject of grace. Grace is a fresh start in each NOW moment. That's how each moment becomes a wow, as in *"wow, you mean no past?!"* Yup. No past. That's what this is, no past, no future, only this now. This spontaneous, universal mind field of cosmic consciousness has no time lag as we experience here in 3D. It happens instantly. For those wanting instant gratification, it doesn't get more instant than this. So . . . that's why we're in training right now. We're getting ready for this by finding out just how it works – with time lag.

Practice makes perfect. As you might expect, this is not going to all happen in the twinkling of an eye. Well actually it will, but we're having a little dry run first. Time is collapsing, as you may have noticed already as things are speeding up towards no time lag and the 5th dimension.

Practice Makes Perfect

Your cells are being infused with light. Your brain patterns are being infused with light. Copious mucous indicates, **shit out, light in.** This sheds a whole new light on the meaning of brain drain.

Consequently sleeping and eating patterns may become topsy turvey. Continuity may slide . . . right out the door. New windows of opportunity open. Sequence and consequence may radically shift.

Don't worry. You may be surprised. You may be flabbergasted. But don't worry.

Focus on what's right about it. Get comfortable with these new ideas as they present themselves to you. Practice seeing what's totally and utterly right about you and what's right for you in whatever is going on. Practice makes perfect.

If you feel a deep inner knowing that you **must** eat junk food, OD on chocolate, snack til you burst, to name just a few of thing's we've experienced, follow that. Follow your spirit and do whatever IT directs. This is the guiding light for the time ahead.

Practice makes perfect.

Crazy, man, CRAZY!

Now, let's talk about crazy. Feelings of being crazy, or going crazy, or things just generally being very very cra–zee. It's true, they are. But there is one thing we'd like very much to assure you of. You are not crazy.

You are also not alone. Millions and millions of us are going through the equivalent of light body puberty. It's awful. It's maddening. It's ridiculous And it's happening! And it certainly helps to know this. You're not wacko or flaky, even if it seems like it.

Also not everyone is going through the same things at the same time. There are some in the avant garde, some in the middle and some who haven't yet heard the news but who will, eventually, bring up the rear.

When in doubt, you can sing along with Bob Marley
". . . everything's gonna be all right now . . . "

LAUGH !

Laughter really IS the best medicine. Laugh at what you used to focus on before you changed to what you're focusing on now. Laughter oxygenates. Did you know that? The more you oxygenate, the better you'll feel, and more quickly too. We are not saying don't cry. Cry. Cry as much as you can. And when that very important and necessary step is done, laugh. Laugh as much as you can.

YAWN ! ! !

Yawning oxygenates. It's also an indicator of your body being able to go interdimensional. And then back to here. And then going interdimensional again. And then back to here again. You're aclimatizing to pass out and pass over. Isn't that interesting? The "sleep" state is too. You go to the other dimensions and then come back to this one here. You collect data there and the body is infused more and more here until slowly, but surely, we find there is Here. Here and Now. So, if you need more "sleep," go for it. If you cannot get out of bed, don't. If you need to become a couch potato and do TV or videos until all hours, do. Follow your spirit, no matter what.

GOOD Grief ?!??! . . .

Now it may be that a lot of grief sweeps through. Perhaps it won't. But, perhaps it will. This is good. Expressing grief is good. See, 3D is about depression, repression and suppression quite a lot. 5D, where we're headed, is about expression. Any repressed and suppressed stuff is like that doo-doo, that brain drain, it's time for it to go. So . . . let it out. Let it go. Don't hang on or put the lid on one more time. Let it go. Weep. Cry. Gnash your teeth. Shout, scream, pound your pillows. Do whatever it is you have to do. But do let it out Then send it down the tunnel and into the light. That's what it wants. It needs your help to do that.

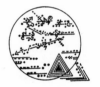

Then, and here's the best part, tonally kiss it goodbye. Make vibrational tonals or tonal language sounds, or gobbledegook style sounds, whatever it takes to express the feelings of loss, grief, anger, fear, sadness, relief, gladness, joy and then delight. As you see, this is a progression of sequences or stages that bring you to the other side, the farther shore or the light side of the tunnel. This is a clearing and a cleansing of thought patterning to speed up that progress.

We found "Aldebaran" and "Emerald" as recommended in the "Starlight Elixirs and Cosmic Vibrational Healing" book (by Michael Smulkis and Fred Rubenfeld, Woodstock, NY: Beekman Publications) to be enormously helpful to our processing of grief. This book and starlight elixirs are available from Pegasus Products, P. O. Box 228, Boulder, CO 80306, 1-800-527-6104, email: starvibe@indra.net.

Detaching From Attachments

If anything matters to you, it materializes. This is a further refinement of focus. Right now on our training programme we're learning how to detach. We're detaching from old things and going for new things. If you're attached, the pain is greater as the attachment is, literally, broken. You see, you can't take it with you. So, give it up gracefully and gratefully. Grateful that you had a time to play. Now is the time to go home to some new toys. This is what the universe is wanting to give you, the next toys to play with. If things matter so much to you that you continue to focus on and materialize them when we're in a dematerializing or counterflow, you get zapped. By going opposite to the flow you get zapped by the molecular spin. It's a new kind of slap in the face. But . . . if this is what it

OVERWHELM !

Anything that looks pretty much like overwhelm, whether physical, mental, or emotional can be benefitted by using a rescue remedy. There are two sorts we've tried. At first we knew only of the Bach Flower Remedy called *Rescue Remedy*. Then we discovered the Pegasus Starlight Elixir called *Zeta Cygni, Starry Rescue*. Take according to your spiritual directions. This may be the time to mention heart palpitations. Heart palpitations generally are caused by two things. Either the heart rate is speeded up for shunting out toxins. Or, your new electrics are coming on line and the heart is shifting to the new beat. But if you are in any doubts, do consult your health practitioner.

ALLOWING . . . is a Technology

One of the most important things to know is this. Let whatever is happening, happen. If you're dreadfully worried, go to your health practitioner. But generally, the transmutation process is a miraculous one. It does its level best to not KO you. By focusing on the miracle which is closer than breathing, you turn it round so everything's OK with you. So, our experience is this. Go wherever "it" wants to take you. By allowing and being open to the process, this becomes quite a journey of discovery. In this journey you may find as we have done, that you can still function even with a raging 3 day old migraine or full montezuma's revenge when you focus on the upside rather than the downside.

Brain Mutation

I have actually experienced going blind on a number of occasions. This is radical and dramatic and it may not ever happen to you. But sometimes when a process is in full swing, it's best to let that complete itself with the least amount of panic. Oxygenate. Breathe. Breathing definitely assists, especially if you stay put. All brains are mutating. So you will have lumps and bumps and sore spots on your skull as the brain expands. The optic nerves are mutating as part of the brain's process. You may have ocular headaches or migraines. Soon you will start seeing multidimensionally and universally. We suggest you do what's best for you to go with this flow. And by the way, the soul enters through the eyes and flows into your cell suit. This is how your soul and spirit fly into the mystical new intergalactic you.

Cell Fire

Cell fire is a burning off process. It affects male and female bodies alike. It is not menopausal or hormonal in and of itself so much as an energetic cleansing, in the same vein as it were, as diarrhea and brain drain. If you are at all worried, do have it checked by your health practitioner.

Don't Stop ! Go ! Go ! Go !

Avoid taking anti-diarrheals, flu or cold remedies or cough medicines. Our advice is not to stop the processes, but let them rip. The body is efficient. Nature is efficient. The universe is efficient. The body takes only whatever time and energy it needs. Allow its wisdom full rein and give this your willing and able cooperation. This facilitates and eliminates a lot of false starts and unnecessary retakes. It harmonizes body and mind with spirit more easily, serenely, gracefully and gratefully when you acknowledge and give your whole-hearted cooperation. You may get discouraged. It's human to do so. We suggest you take the road less travelled and just keep on keepin' on.

Trust . . . is a Technology

Apart from physical body clearing, there is also mental body clearing and emotional body clearing going on. Old thought patterns, old emotional patterns, old reactions, a lot of old stuff in general is now coming up for review and release into the light. Like we said before, you can't take it with you.

Because we are in human body transmitter-receivers, most of the stuff we may pick up on the airwaves is the general human outpouring at this time. Vibrationally, they may seem yours. But mostly they are not. Thoughts and emotions spread vibrationally. You know very well how someone's anger hits you in the stomach. The same is true for thoughts and feelings. This particular thing took us years to really get a handle on. But now we know when things are not ours, so we simply don't identify with them as ours. A lot of self-reproach and judgement can be avoided. But what cannot be avoided is knowing what your job is. Whatever comes to you, comes to you because your job is to clear it because you have both the knowhow and the wherewithall to do so. "It" knows that.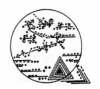

So, we vow break, do tunnel vision, scream, cry, do tonals or whatever is required to effect "its" expression and release into the light. You can do the same. It's not personal you see, it's transpersonal. We can each help clear up this old stuff by being an open channel for its transfiguration and transubstantiation too. The faster the better, as far as we're concerned.

So trust is a technology. When you act on faith and take each leap of faith as it presents itself, it becomes your new automatic pilot. It steers you out of the abyss and into bliss. Trust us. We know whereof we speak.

Breathing . . . is a Technology

You can trigger yourself into a calm, relaxed or altered state very simply. Anywhere. Any time. It works like this :

- using the diaphragm breathing method where your abdomen expands as you breathe in, breath in to a slow count of 7
- hold that breath to a slow count of 7
- breathe out to a slow count of 7 expelling the air through the mouth as the abdomen retracts towards the spine
- hold to a slow count of 7
- do this 7 times
- on the last exhalation, count down from 7 to 1 and then ask your body and your life field to **relax**. Hold that **relax** feeling during the final hold to a slow count of 7. Then breathe normally for a couple of breaths.

This needs only a little practice for you to experience that you are easily able to switch into **relax** mode and that you can flick it on like a light switch, just like that.

This is a wonderful technique for banishing 4AM heebie jeebies and getting some sleep! It also works for panic attacks or sudden onset anxiety in traffic jams, shopping malls or other public emotional jams and mental gridlocks. When you relax, the vibration spreads, and all relax. Try it. You'll breathe a lot easier for it.

Watch little kids. They breathe this way normally. You did too, once. Through a bit of focus and practice, you can return to this natural and normal breathing mode too.

Sing. Out loud. Ever notice how singers breathe? You know the words to so many songs. Sing them. *"Every step you take, every move you make, every breath you take . . . "*

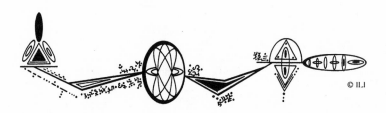

© ILI

IV. Let There Be Light, and There IS Light

Imagine for a moment that you are in another dimension. You're doing your utmost to assist the human beings in this dimension who are shape shifting and shit shifting. The differences between the two dimensions, or these two different worlds is hard to bridge. So you try out a few things. Maybe you remember Patrick Swayze and all the things he tried in order to get "through" to Demi Moore in the movie *"Ghost."* He was in one dimension and she and Tony "the rat" Goldwyn were in another. As she becomes more and more open to the possibilities of contacting him, as her love carries her through all the crazy stuff going down, she and he can meet. Their two different worlds meet. It's beautiful. It's touching. It's joyful. It's inspiring. It's drenched through and through with luminous love and luminous light. You feel it and you're set a–light too.

This is an experience. How can you possibly hope to describe this to someone? They have to experience it for themselves.

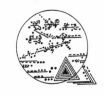

So this is what the other dimensional teams are doing. They're presenting lots and lots of ways so we can feel how this different world feels. Intellectualizations do not feel. Intellectual mode is built to categorize and dismiss. It is not built to feel. Just like Demi Moore, our job is to entertain the possibilities. You can be open to things which may just seem plain crazy, when there's this feeling, that "something tells me" sort of thing. Nothing ventured nothing gained, as they say.

Thoughts such as "I can't!" may come up. If so, remember this. Thoughts are just thoughts. Just because you have them doesn't mean they're real. Thoughts happen. Thinking happens. But just because it happens doesn't make it real. It's just something happening. You can still have these thoughts and act on faith. You can still take your leap of faith. And another thing you can do is to take all those "I can'ts" into the tunnel and bust their little butts. Send them into the light. Their job's over. Your job's just beginning. This is the training programme, remember? Co-creating with the light. No worries. No problemo, you say. Let there be light.

And there IS light.

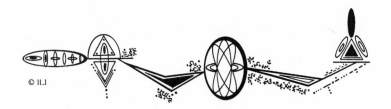

© ILI

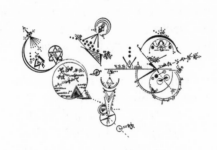

Glimpses
Into
The
Invisible

•

Tools and
Resources to
Begin Working
With Your Own
Energy Medicine
for the
New Millennium

•

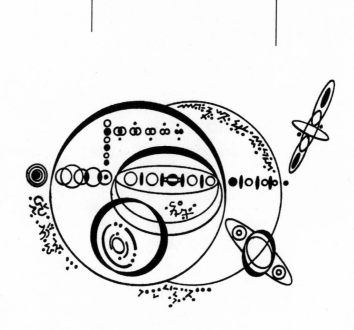

Glimpses into the Invisible Worlds

The world is speeding up, there is no doubt about that. In Einsteinian physics it is a given that processes speed up towards their end. It is also readily apparent to many that we are, indeed, approaching the end of this world as we've known it. Soon the world is going to be a very different place. Everyone in one way or another can just feel it. The only thing about it is that we just won't know how different it will be, until we're actually there.

In the meanwhile, here we are in the midst of shifting ground rules for living on planet Earth. We are simply inundated with more information than we can ever possibly comprehend. Health issues in our increasingly polluted world are of paramount importance. Yet the information is far too often conflicting and contradictory. In a technologically accelerated society, we feel increasingly alienated and disconnected not only from the basics of Life, but from the sacredness of our lives. Thus we become out of balance with Nature and with Life and physically, mentally, emotionally and spiritually sick. Buildings, food, clothing, water, medications, electronic pollution and more, all contribute to our sickness. We are increasingly aware of our lack of purpose and are searching for ways to wake up and pierce through the veils of illusion.

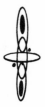

In our view, these and many other "negatives" which have become our daily norm, present us with grand possibilities. These "negative alarms" which are going off are also serving to awaken us to new possibilities. For those waking up to the unseen and the unknown, there are many tools for your little invisible tool box. We present you with some of them in the following pages. We've tested them out for ourselves and include them here as new *toys* with which you can experiment. You can experiment in reading and working with energies and you can experience how energy moves and positively or negatively affects your life. This is the start of energy medicine. The guidance for using it comes from within. It's called in-tuition.

We are spirit incarnate in a physical body and we are mastering the techniques that bridge these two differing parts of ourselves into a happier, more integrated and higher quality of life. Intuition and inner knowing then unfold our present little glimpses into the so-called invisible worlds into vast new vistas into which we can then walk and take our rightful place.

TransFiguration Chakra Balancer

The Universe is a powerful Life Energy Field. Our visible world is surrounded by a far vaster invisible world. Indeed, our visible world is only about 2% visible matter and the other 98% of our bodies, furniture, animals, trees, planet and our universe is composed of invisible space. Our visible world is, actually, frozen light. The invisible worlds of space are full of fast moving energy or light waves. We can capture these light waves by "freeze framing" their patterns. This is called a yantra, or the frequency pattern of a higher vibration which has been captured and pictorialized. It is a sacred or holy thing simply because certain patterns contain the power to imprint our bodies with their life waves. This gets us *moving,* in concert with them. Moving energy is healthy energy. Stuck or slow energy is unhealthy energy.

The healing pattern of the **TransFiguration Chakra Balancer** is a template through which healing energies can travel into our 98% space and resonate our material bodies into an upward shift. The body is shifted upwardly into harmonic resonance with the healing pattern.

This new artform symbology work comes from Higher Orders in service to Earth and those who feel drawn to work with them.

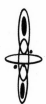

Zon-O-Ray is a completely intuitive artist. Like me, she has spent the last ten years "in training" to Inner Guidance in order to be of service to others on this spiritual journey of self-discovery and self-actualization.

The Chakra Balancer functions as an energy anchor. It supports your physical, mental, emotional and spiritual alignment into At-one-ment. It can be used to charge, or imprint your food and water with healing and purifying frequencies. It can also be used to *discharge* low vibrational frequencies out of your bed and body, and your living and working spaces. These are the spaces and places where you spend the most time and can be the most adversely affected by low-lying and psychic debris and stuck energy patterns which cause you to go round and round in circles.

Each person is unique and will be able to feel, read and play with energies differently. There is no right way. Like yoga, there is also no comparison nor competition. You do and feel what is simply yours to do and feel.

Here are some suggested guidelines, however, to get you started on your journey of self-realization and self-actualization:
- meditate with it
- sleep with it under your mattress or pillow
- use it as a place mat to infuse your food and water or juices with chi, especially for the ill or elderly
- it acts as a high energy enhancer for any food or water in your kitchen or in your fridge
- lay it on particular chakras on either the front or back of your body
- use it in bodywork or any healing work you do with others

• hang it on the wall to infuse your living or work area. It acts as a doorway, infusing yourself and others with higher energy medicine frequencies over longer periods of time.

It is easy to recharge and cleanse the **TransFiguration Chakra Balancer** by simply wiping it clean and laying it in the sun for a few minutes. In energy work, it's important to do this often.

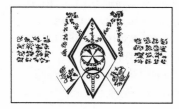

The **TransFiguration Chakra Balancer** is an 11 inch (28 cm) by 17 inch (43 cm) laminated card. The symbology designs on it come in three colors :
magenta, purple and sky blue.

Please allow your intuition to choose the correct color ray or frequency which is best for you.

The TransFiguration Chakra Balancer costs $30. Please write or email for shipping & handling charges.

Please make checks or money orders payable and send to:
InterDimensional Light Infusions
PMB 172 • 2370 W. Hwy 89A, #11 • Sedona, AZ 86336-5349 • USA
E–mail: zzlights@hotmail.com

InterDimensional Light Infusions

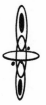

Private Readings, Sacred Art and Sacred Spaces

Private readings are transmissions from higher levels of Self and like all of Zon-O-Ray's art, are called **InterDimensional Light Infusions**. A reading is unique to each individual. Zon-O-Ray has the unique ability to tune into each individual's highest energy field of Self and translate their subtle energies from the invisible into this dimension's visible domain. She uses specific colors and artform symbologies from the causal energy body to infuse the 98% of space within your physical body on this plane.

This private reading can thus enhance the release of psychic debris and low level thoughtforms from your auric field, leading to self-healing when combined with the other energy medicine light work encapsulated in this book.

All that is required is your permission, your name, address and phone number and your date of birth. It is preferable, but not necessary, to provide your sun sign along with your moon and ascendant.

The cost is $175 for an 11 inch (28 cm) by 17 inch (43 cm) artwork which is then laminated so that it can be used for the light infusion of your food, your body and your working or living space etc.

In addition, larger scale artwork pieces and also altar pieces can be commissioned for light infusion work in sacred spaces in homes and offices, especially in conjunction with Feng Shui. Altars can be made for your own deities or those which Zon-O-Ray can provide for you.

If you'd like more information about enhancing the sacredness of your life on this plane, a full color brochure is available upon request from the address above.

The Chi Machine

Although I am not a real fan of most machines, this particular machine delivers a chi rush of healing energy which is most exciting to actually feel. Oxygen plus chi make you feel *high*. If you've never really experienced cosmic chi energy running through and around your body before, then you are in for a very wonderful experience. Your feet are positioned on the machine and they swing from side to side. This *swimming fish* action decompressess the spine and oxygenates the body with absolutely no effort on your part. It's a **lying down exercise. Isn't that great!** Detox is combined with organ massage to flush toxins rapidly out of the body. So you drink pure water before and after the exercise to carry waste products away.

Zon-O-Ray and I meditate while on the machine. We've both experienced deep relaxation as well as peak moments of inspiration and insight via the altered states we enter. I have had a very bad back for years which the Chi Machine has now eliminated, along with expensive monthly chiropractic bills. Other people have reported benefits in their own unique and widely differing ways. Energy medicine is specific to each person's needs and make-up. Each person will heal, or become whole in their return to One-ness, differently.

The **Sun Harmony Chi Machine** is the culmination of some 38 years of research by Dr. Inoue of Japan. As head of the *Japanese Oxygen Association* he was searching for the perfect way to maximally, but simply, oxygenate the body. As you would expect, there are several "copy cat" machines on the market now, but their cheaper mechanisms can harm your back.

The Chi Machine is certainly a rather expensive investment at $460 plus shipping and handling. However there is a 14 day money back guarantee just in case you may not be completely satisfied. Should you be interested, we'll send you an information pack. The machine is not available through shops but only through sales by individuals. In addition, the Chi Machine is compatible with any of the various electrical systems around the world.

InterDimensional Light Infusions
PMB 172 • 2370 W. Hwy 89A, #11
Sedona, AZ 86336-5349 • USA
E–mail: zzlights@hotmail.com

o

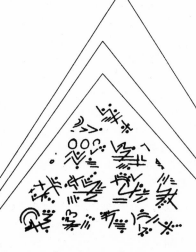

We emphasize that our great love is to move forward and that this is our first "go" at transmitting in this form. We hope you find as much joy and delight in it as we have done at getting it to this, our first stage of public presentation here on Earth.

An Invitation to the Cosmic Dance

We, the Infinite Life Forms of this manifest and unmanifest Creation request the pleasure of your company to join us in taking the next steps in the journey home to Source.

The appointed Time and Place in your Space is Now.

This vast and magnificent event unfolding across Creation is now unfolding in your dimension, on your planet, and within you.

We intend to dance the night away. You're invited.

Let's Dance!

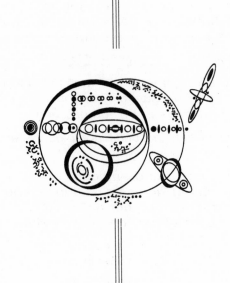

Index

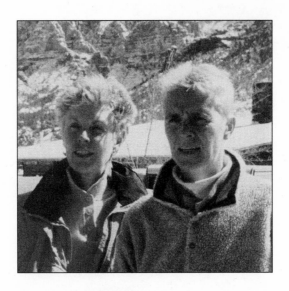

You might like to know a little about Zon-O-Ray and zho-de-Rah
who've put this book together.

They have absolutely no earthly degrees, qualifications or
references for doing so.
They source from off-planet
making the data they find there
as relevant as possible
to this planet here.

They are here to **re**–member their family and friends
in the only way they know how —
by making new waves.
The ripple effect is a quickening.
The slip stream a guide
to the times
ahead.